THE LIFE AND DEMISE OF NORMAN CAMPBELL

1909 to 2012

The autobiography of Norman Campbell
An ordinary man who tells his story at the extraordinary
age of 103

THE LIFE AND DEMISE OF NORMAN CAMPBELL

or

A VERY SILVER SURFER
@ 102

or

TO THE END OF THE WORLD
AND BACK AGAIN
'Just because I could'

or

Norman's tells his own story

compiled by

Diana Jackson

EVENTISPRESS

©2013

Diana Jackson

Norman Campbell's life story is true to his amazing memory.

A CIP catalogue record for this title
is available from the British Library

ISBN : 978-0-9572520-6-6

First Published in 2013

Published by Eventispress
Bedford
UK
www.eventispress.co.uk

Printed by CreateSpace

Dedication

To Mae and Peggy

Acknowledgements

Thanks to all of Norman's extended family who have given him so much pleasure over the years and have agreed to be mentioned in this autobiography.

Thanks to the Kingston Archives who have helped with photos and newspaper resources and to The Surrey Comet for giving permission to print adverts and articles from 1911 to 1912.

Thanks to Norman himself. It has been a pleasure to spend time with him as he has shared his vast and wonderful memories. This book, Norman's memoirs, is also illustrated by photos and pictures from his multitude of albums and scrap books, squirreled away over more than a century.

Forward

I HAVE HAD the pleasure of knowing Norman all of my life, in fact I'm told that he came to my christening in Warlingham, Surrey. For years I knew him as Mr Campbell and each Sunday, if the sun shone, my mum would say,

'I expect Mr and Mrs Campbell will pop over,' and invariably they did.

I remember them sharing our Christmases right up until when I went to college, at about the same time as Mrs Campbell, Norman's first wife Peggy, passed away.

As Norman reached 100 he shared many snippets of his life with us and in the past year it has been a privilege for me to listen to his full life story.

Norman has lived through both World Wars; he vividly remembers the transition from horse drawn vehicle to the motor car, the technological advances of radio, cinema and record production and he sees himself as a pioneer, for example, in television ownership.

It is a fascinating tale, including Norman's journey to Australia in the late 20's, but he also describes his various job roles from working in service as a lad out of school. through many transformations until his final post in Decca, where he witnessed first-hand the development of gramophone records.

His personal life is full of humour, alongside key poignant memories and I believe that Norman has shared with me many secrets, which he has not divulged in years.

As he talked of rediscovering his childhood sweetheart Mae late in life, he gained not only a wonderful lady, with whom he shared many happy years, but also a whole new family, who have been a life line to him, especially in his last years.

Still alert, with a sharp mind and clear recollection of dates, events and adventures in his life, even at 102 years of age, Norman tells his own story in his own words, transcribed from a series of interviews videoed over several months.

I saw Norman in hospital three days before he passed away and he said,
    'I've got it Diana! The name of my book.
    'The Life and Demise of Norman Campbell!'
    'You can't call it that,' I spluttered. 'You're still with us.'

By Diana Jackson

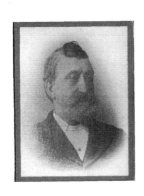

Grandad William Campbell

Grandmother Eliza Campbell

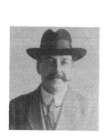

Norman's Father Spencer

Norman's Mother Annie (Matthews)

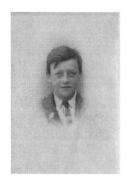

Norman Spencer Campbell

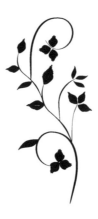

Sister Vera Gladys Campbell

CHAPTER 1

Norman Campbell's
Early Years
You are a Hampshire Hog!

1909

I WAS BORN in Bishopstoke, Eastleigh, Hampshire in 1909. My mother used to say,

'You are a Hampshire Hog.[1]'

I've no idea why she called me that but it was on 4th October 1909 that I was born.

My father worked on the railway. His father was a foreman at Nine Elms railway depot at Battersea, where they built railway engines, and all the male members of the family started serving their apprenticeship there.

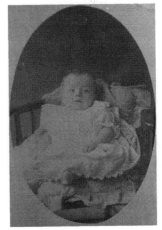

When my Dad got married they moved to Eastleigh because they had opened another depot to build the locomotives down there.

My mother sang and my father played the piano. They were often invited to parties and she used to do the singing and he used to do the playing. That's how they came together and got married and that's how it all started.

1. There is no real record of the origin of Hampshire Hog

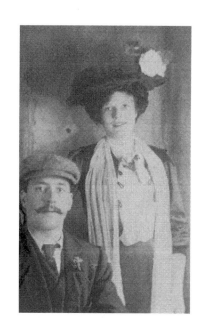

Spencer and Annie Campbell

Back up to London

1911

WE DIDN'T STAY in Eastleigh very long, but came back to London and finished up in Norwood. Dad left his job because it was heavy work building railway engines using cranes to lift the shafts on to the wheels and this was just when the automobile had started to come in.

He said he'd get into motor cars, because they were always hand built in those days and it was easier to assemble the gear box on a bench than it was lugging all those railway parts about. So he got into Autocarriers[2] at Norwood and they decided to shift down to Thames Ditton and that's how we came to get in this very house in 1911 when I was two years old.

Dad was in and out of work and I remember a lot of times when we were broke, but there were no human rights like there is today and they would say,
'We haven't got enough work. We'll lay you off for a week and then we'll call you back.'
Then they might work for three days and then be laid off again, just like that.

2.   Autocarriers Limited was formed by John Portwine in 1904 and moved to Ferry Works, Thames Ditton in 1911, extending its range of mainly business vehicles to light cars. By 1922 AC racing cars were seen driven at nearby Brooklands and at Monte Carlo.

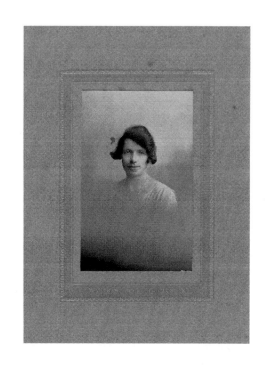

Annie ~ Norman's Mother

MY MUM WAS a lovely woman. Her hair was long and black. She was a bit of a clairvoyant. She used to dream of the future and tell fortunes with the cards and tea leaves and that sort of thing and the neighbours hung on to her every word. She used to believe in it all and that something would turn the corner one day, but it never did. Not for her anyway.

That's why I feel guilty sometimes. I've come into all of it and they had nothing. She'd be pleased for me though; of course she would.

There was another thing. My mother was dead scared of mice. One morning a mouse came out of the firebox. She screamed in fright and pulled her skirts up around her. (Norman laughed)

Mind you I had a very happy childhood. There were no rows or anything like that.

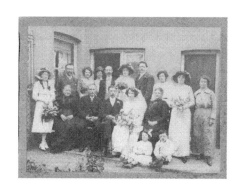

A family Wedding — Aunt Ethel married Harry Hedge
Norman is sitting with his sister Vera at the front

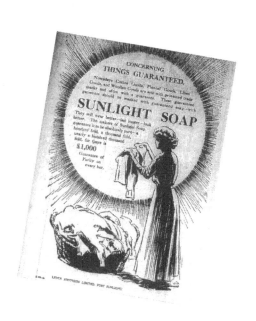

Over 100 Years of Life at Home

1911 – 2011.......

THIS WAS THE scullery where I have the kitchen today. Over in that corner was the copper where the washing was done every Monday morning and there was a fire underneath. We'd do the rinsing outside with the mangle. Then on Tuesday it used to be ironing and folding and putting away.

There was a sink half way along the wall. It wasn't a very deep sink and it was always awash with water, about six inches. There was one tap for all of the house where we had to wash ourselves too. Everything had to be done at that sink.

Then there was a little table next to the sink and a gas stove in the other corner over there. We came here in 1911 and, between 1912 to 1914, they got a gas stove.

Opposite, I remember there used to be a couple of bikes. There were duck boards down on the floor and the floor was always wet, I remember that. well.

You can see the outside loo through the window even now, but then it was free standing. Of course, since then I've enclosed it in the conservatory and so it's all indoors now.

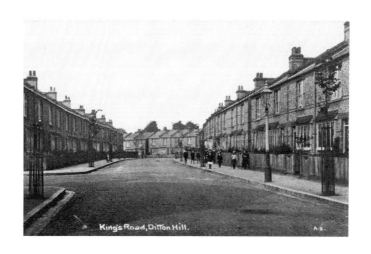

Kings Road Ditton Hill

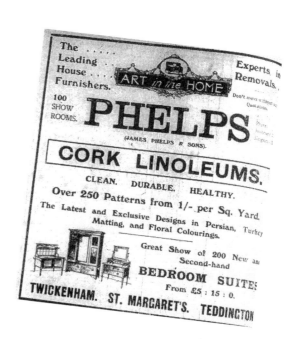

In the back room there was a high shelf and a kitchen range set back into the fireplace. We got all the heat for the house from there in those days, but we have the gas fire now. There was an oven on one side and a hob on the top, where you could have a kettle steaming away all day for cups of tea.

This was the main room we lived in. There wasn't much furniture, only a table, four chairs, a couch along the wall and a dresser next to the fireplace with shelves up to the ceiling and I've still got the base out in the conservatory. On the other side of the range there was a food cupboard.

We had lino on the floor in here in those days. It was imitation stuff and you had to be very careful because it would tear easily. My mother used to make rag rugs. She'd get hessian and old clothes, which she cut into strips, and she thread them through the hessian, pushing them with a bodger, which had a little lever on it and a sharp end. When I was getting older it used to be one of my jobs on a Saturday morning to go and shake all the rugs out in the garden.

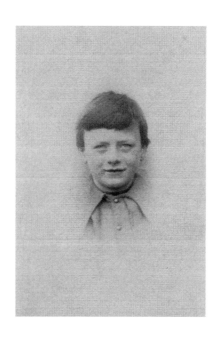

Young Norman

Under the stairs was the coal cellar in those days. You could still find coal dust down there today but I've put a bit of carpet over it now. The coal man used to come in here with the coal on his back and that's where he used to shoot the coal. All the dust would fly up in the hall. Schewww! You can imagine.

Most people have taken this cupboard out to give more room and maybe have a telephone or something under the stairs. I have filled in the banisters though, and put in a false ceiling because it was far too high up to paper.

In the front room we had a glass cabinet with lots of ornaments and a piano with music on it near the widow and a piano stool. My father used to play by ear. He couldn't read music but when he was in lodgings he used to tinker about and he taught himself to play. He was always a quick learner like me.

We had three bedrooms upstairs in those early days. Of course there was no sink, in fact there was no bathroom at all: just the one tap in the scullery. The only difference to today is that we've now only got two bedrooms because we put the bathroom in the other bedroom in 1956.

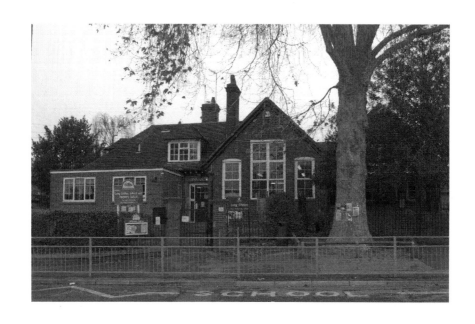

Norman's Primary School as it looks today

CHAPTER 2

Memories of School Days and the start of World War One

1914

I WENT TO Ditton Hill Primary School at five years old, just across the road, and we used to get there through the alleyway. There were four classrooms and I was in the baby's one to start with; Class 1 and we had a Headteacher whose name was Mrs Nettle and my teacher's name was Miss Passey.

I used to say to my Mum, 'Can I bring my teacher home to tea?'
Of course Mum said, 'yes,' but Mrs Passey never came.

We had a May Pole and my partner's name was Doris Way. One day we did some painting and I was told to bring in a flower, so I took in a bluebell, but I finished up with a big blue blob.
The teacher said, 'That's nothing like a bluebell!'

I can always see that big blob of blue. (Norman chuckled)

The other thing I remember was when we had a doctor and a nurse and they used to come around and look through your head for nits with a knitting needle. I suppose I must have had this sour expression on my face and the doctor said,
'Here you are son, here's a penny. Get yourself a penny's worth of laughter.'

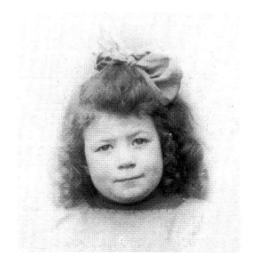

Young Sister Vera

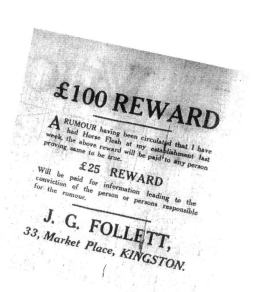

£100 REWARD

A RUMOUR having been circulated that I have
had Horse Flesh at my establishment last
week the above reward will be paid to any person
proving same to be true.

£25 REWARD

Will be paid for information leading to the
conviction of the person or persons responsible
for the rumour.

J. G. FOLLETT,
33, Market Place, KINGSTON.

I remember my mother was pushing my sister in a pram once and a woman came up to us and said, ' the war's broken out!'

Then one day my mother took me over to Kingston and said,' Try this out. It's flag butter.'
There were two flags crossed on it and of course it was margarine, because butter was very expensive in the war.

My father was a charge hand at the munitions factory during the First World War. All the factories like Auto Carriers were now doing war work. He'd work a fortnight on days and a fortnight on nights; a twenty four hour operation you see, to keep the war going.

I don't remember much about World War 1 because I was only five, but on a Monday they still had a cattle market over there in Kingston. There were pounds where they put the sheep in the pens and I remember a butcher called Folletts because we used to have a saveloy in a roll for our dinner while we sat to watch the sheep and hens.

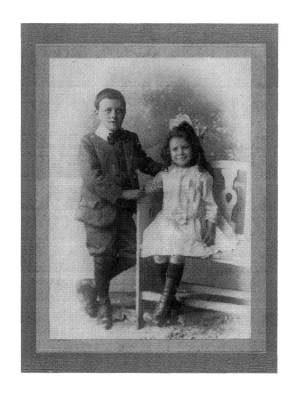

Norman and his sister Vera
Norman was about eight at the time

1917

When I was eight years old I went to the bigger school. The first school master's name was Mr Mileham. There was this particular Monday morning when I said to my mother, 'I don't feel well.'

I think I was trying to get off school because I didn't feel like going in that day so she said, 'Best get back to bed then.'

At about half past nine I heard all this noise outside my bedroom window and there was a crowd of children coming up the road.

I poked my head out the window and said, 'What's up?'

They shouted back, 'Mileham's committed suicide. We've got the day off!' So of course I felt better then, all of a sudden, and I was up and out with them. I remember that.

I was too young to worry about what had happened to Mr Mileham. Maybe it was the war but it's funny how a child reacts if you think about it. I was just pleased to have time off school.

The next Headmaster they nicknamed Bouncer because he used to bounce about and his wife taught us too, but he was always away doing something. He would gad about and she used to take the two classes actually. He started up a football team and took the lads out to the recreation ground to run.

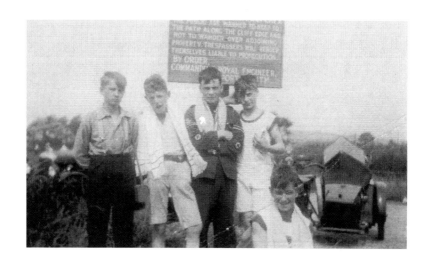

Norman and friends

One day we set off running, but soon he shouted out to me,

'You can't run fast enough.'

So that was the end of my football career. Believe it or not he had an AC car, that's a two seater with a Dickey, a seat in the boot which you pulled down to give an extra seat.

He transported the whole team, that's eleven kids in this two seater! They didn't go far though, to Tolworth or somewhere local. There were two in the back and two in the front, that's four. Then they had kids clinging on to the running board on either side. Eleven kids. That's unbelievable.

The road outside this house was more like a playground with about fifty kids playing and we'd have different seasons. We'd have hoops and skipping ropes in the summer and cigarette cards and marbles.

Then in the winter we used to have a winter warmer; tin cans filled with oily rags and we'd set alight to them and they'd flare away.

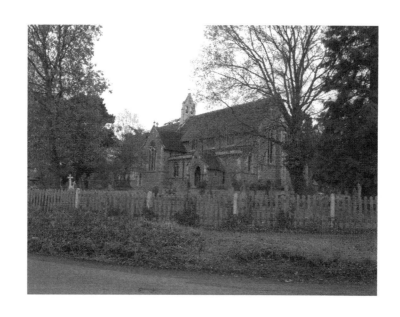

St Mary's Church Long Ditton

CHAPTER 3

Norman's Early Memories of Church

Get behind me Satan!
And he got behind me!

I ALSO REMEMBER, when I was about eight years old, the vicar got up to the lectern one day and said,

'Thou shalt not kill.'

And the next time he was saying,

'Pick up thy sword and slay thine enemy.'

I thought, what's this all about? It didn't make much sense to me. People believe in it and they get solace from it but I've never believed. I've got through to 102 and it never helped me in anyway. I'm afraid you've got to have religion to keep law and order, to put the fear of God in people, and it did in those days.

When I was growing up you heard more about the bloke down below. That put the fear of God in us if nothing else.

'Satan will have you, that's where you'll go, burning in fire,' and all that sort of preaching.

'Oooh,' you said, 'that's not a place for me to go.'

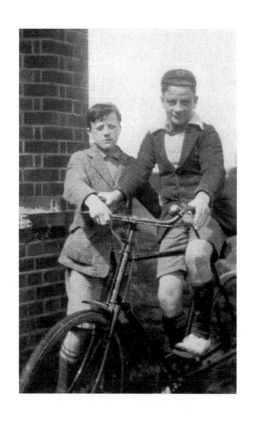

Sunday afternoons

Another funny story was about a little boy who lived up the road; his name was Aubrey. He got caught nicking something, an apple probably, and the minister said,

'Aubrey, you shouldn't do that. You shouldn't take anything and if you think you are going to do it again then you must say to yourself,

Get behind me Satan.'

Aubrey told us that next time he fancied an apple he said to himself,

'Get behind me Satan,'

But Satan said, 'You take it Aubrey.'

Well. (Norman laughed, his shoulders shaking and his eyes lit up with the memory) What do you think of that? A bright kid though. I always remember that.

We went to church sometimes three times a Sunday; once in church and sometimes to Sunday school, then we had a bible class on Sunday afternoons and then church in the evening. We always had Sunday lunch and Sunday tea and the church bells would ring for the evening service at half past six. When I was about fourteen, in the afternoon we'd stroll around and get up to mischief at Tolworth, Molesey or Thames Ditton, looking for the girls.

We used to have some fun in those days.

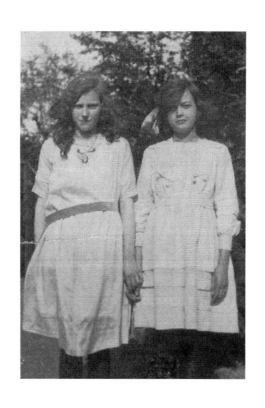

Mae aged about fourteen years
On the right

CHAPTER 4

There I go Meeting Mae

1920

I MET MAE when we were at school. In those days the kids used to pair you up. I don't know why it happened. I simply got paired up with Mae when I was about eleven and at playtime, if it was a bit cold, we used to go into the classroom and stand around the fire, because there was a big fire in the corner. It was all the heat we had and we used to lean on the guard and chat away. It just seemed to gel between us.

Mae lived across the road from me but I didn't see her very often, although I saw her going to and coming home from school. I didn't walk her home because I was with all the boys of course, but I just used to see her over the road playing hopscotch, or something like that, and it just went on from there. It gelled as if that was how it should be.

On Sundays we had to go to church and if I sat behind her I used to pull her hair. We got black looks by what'shisname, the vicar, and sometimes told to keep quiet.

Then one day she said,
    'Tonight I'll be up at the window and we can have a chat.'

The effort she must have made to get to that front window; you see, her Mum and Dad were downstairs and she must have crept through and up the stairs and she'd be out there talking to me for half an hour across the street.

My, what a girl!

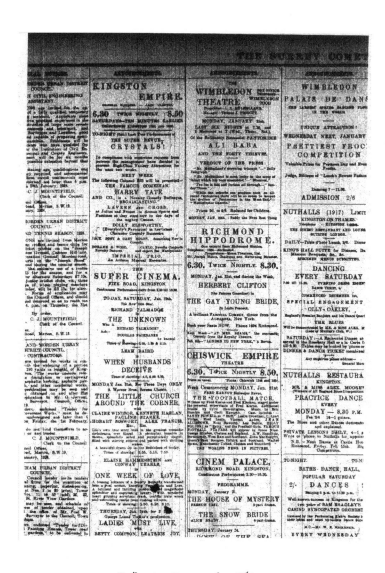

What's On at the Flicks
Surrey Comet

In the early 20's when I was growing up, all our entertainment was the gramophone or people played instruments like the violin, piano and the cornet and you made your own amusement. There were parties and you might take a bottle and have a good time.

In about 1920 there used to be a Saturday morning Penny Cinema for kids called the Cinema Palace or Kinema. We used to go to the silent movies before I went to Australia. They were terrible. They used to have running sagas and they'd go on for about fifteen weeks and I remember one where you had a lead person called Pearl and after an episode of fifteen to twenty minutes it used to end with her tied to the railway. You had to come back next week to see if she was run over and that sort of thing.

In those days they used to have a piano playing music to suit the scene on the movie (de de dela, de de de la, de de de lal la la la....) and sometimes people made sound effects from the side of the stage. It's funny looking back now.

The cinemas in those days were the Kinema, The Cinema Palace and The Super Cinema. These were the Flea Pits; dirty places which we travelled to on the number 73 tram.

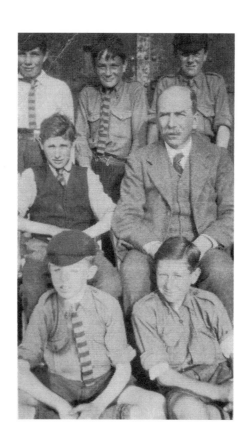

Mr Clayton and the Church Lads' Brigade

CHAPTER 5

Happy Days with the Church Lads' Brigade

1921

I WENT TO that school until I was twelve and a half but I used to belong to the Church Lads Brigade too. All the kids around here belonged. In fact the whole village revolved around the church, even the school. On Sundays you dressed up and walked about and didn't do anything.

It was Mr Clayton, the London solicitor who sent me off to business school. He was the head man around here and he tried to keep all the boys off the street. He opened his big old house up to everybody. It was called the Elms down at the bottom near Rectory Lane but it's not there anymore. They've built about ten houses on the land now.

This site here was one big area and the land belonged to Ditton House. The one over the back was Saxonbury House which joined this one and down the main road there was another house; I can't remember its name. Then you have the pub, The Plough and Harrow in the middle, and then all the other block belonged to the Elms. The school was built on the same grounds. They built 79 houses in Kings Road. There were only 79 because you came to the Saxonbury boundary and there were four houses near there which were bombed during World War 2.

Mr Clayton was a bald headed man with a moustache and glasses and he had a little impediment in his speech. He worked in the family's firm of solicitors at Gower Street. He was quite a nice fellow, but I was one of his favourites. We used to go over to his house of an evening. We could read from his library, play the piano or gramophones or just chat amongst ourselves in his house.

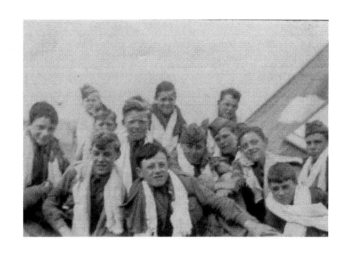

Camping with the Church Lads' Brigade

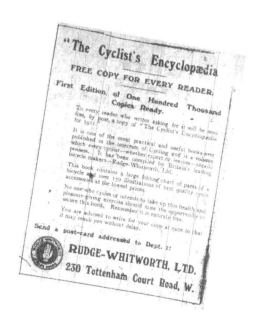

We had a kind of little youth club. At nine o'clock he went to have his supper and he used to say,

'Home!' to all the boys, gesticulating with his hands, but some of us could stay. I used to keep the books for him. I don't think we would pay, but I think it was donations from local people.

You had to be ten before you could join and once this little boy came up, Geoffrey I think he was, and he said,

'Please sir can I join. I'm nine and three quarters and ten in May Sir.'

Mr Clayton replied, 'No you can't lad, not until you're ten.'

It's funny that you remember things like that.

My best friend at big school was Jonny Ovingdon. We were pals, but when I was ten his father, who was a window cleaner, moved down to relations in Dover, so I lost my little friend. I was pally with all the lads of my age up the street though.

Sometimes we went camping at Chalk Quarry near Boxhill with the Lads Brigade and we collected chalk, making little carvings with it which we painted. On other Saturdays Mr Clayton used to say,

'Go down to Mr Nunn's and hire a bike for half a crown,' and he always paid for that, so we went for a cycle ride around the Surrey hills. One Saturday, when we were sitting down beside the road talking, he asked me,

'What do you want to do when you grow up and leave school, Norman?'

I said, 'I don't know,' because in those days there was only the army, navy and air force or going abroad. There were no opportunities except the police force too, I suppose. I didn't want to be a tram driver, bus driver or postman either. Of course everyone wanted to drive a steam engine.

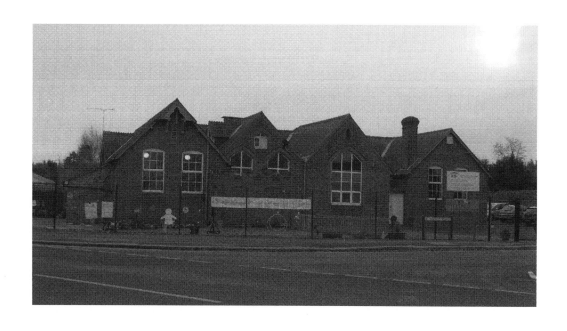

Norman's Secondary School is
Now a Nursery School

I had big ideas and so I said,

'I think I'd like to work up town, in an office. You know, with a bowler hat, striped trousers, black jacket, rolled umbrella and brief case.'
I wanted to look posh going to work up in London.

'Anyway,' he said. 'If that's what you want, I'll send you to Clarks College for a business education; type writing, shorthand and bookkeeping.'

When we left school Mae went into service. All the girls went into service in those days and she was over to Wimbledon. She used to get half a day off a fortnight on a Wednesday to come and see her family and sometimes we met in the street and had a laugh and a giggle and that sort of thing. She had to be in by seven though, but I had a free rein. Unfortunately I didn't see much of her really.

She was pally with another girl Katy and I went out with the boys. We often got on our bikes and went up to Claygate and Molesey to see the girls and this Katy Wootton she said to Mae one day,

'That Norman's been going up seeing girls in the woods,' and that put the boot in at the time, didn't it.

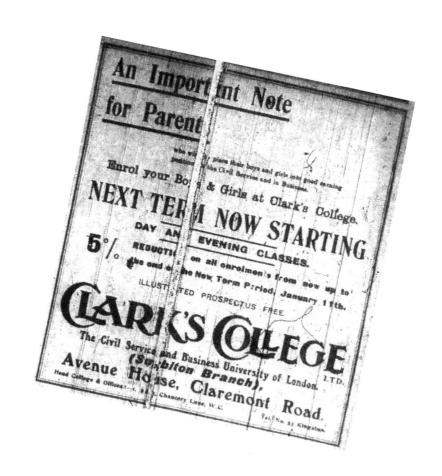

The Surrey Comet

CHAPTER 6

A Man in a Bowler Hat!

1924

I WENT TO Clarke's College for two and a half years and left there at fifteen.

Then Mr Clayton said, 'What are you going to do now?'

I replied, 'I don't know.'

He said, 'The best thing is to put an advert in the paper.'

So we put one in the Comet and there was one reply down at Surbiton, but when I went there it really didn't suit me so then I took a dive down. I was fed up.

Next Mr Clayton said,' There's Don Martin; he's a house boy up at my father's house and he's leaving to go down to Cobham. Would you like to take that on?'

Well, that was a bit of a come down to working in the city; a house boy! I decided I might as well go and so I did that for a little while, working at Hillside House but I didn't care much for it, although I did get the running of the house.

The cook was the governor. She ran everything and controlled the community. I had to get there early in the morning but I was always late. One of my first jobs was to light the boiler. At the start of the day we'd have a cup of tea and she'd say,

'What would you like? Would you care for India or China tea?'
Blimey, I'd never had an offer like that before. That's the first and last time I've ever tasted China tea. I was late a couple of mornings and she got on to me and anyway I thought, I can't stand this, so I put an advert in the national newspaper and to my surprise I got three replies.

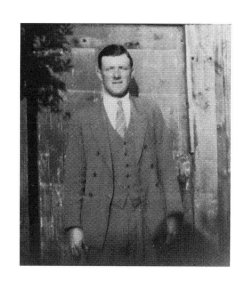

My Office Days

I remember it was thick fog the day I went to look for a job. You couldn't see your hand in front of you. It was terrible. I went to one place and I couldn't find anybody in and so a man said,

> 'I wouldn't go there mate. He's a bit of a shyster.'

He warned me that the man was a moneylender so I took off and never went back there.

Then I went to this other place but their vacancy was filled and so I went up to Fenchurch Street, 4 Lloyd's Avenue, and I got this job for fifteen shillings a week at Cowley and Company. It was fifteen shillings for the fare and so I was just paying for the fare and getting nothing else. Oh dear, my Mother wasn't too pleased.

It was an import and export firm; most of it was sausage skins and they put 300 skins into each barrel. This company sold these skins on the phone and down at the docks.

My job was to bring a sample from the docks and parcel it off to Germany and other places; in fact all over the continent. At the docks there was an atmosphere and smell you can't describe. You'd have to be there. There were all these tunnels under the arches and the smell of the food was everywhere.

The other thing I remember is that I went to the docks at Tower Bridge and on each side of the road there was a man with a cart and a shovel, shovelling up horse manure because of the mess made by all the horse drawn vehicles going about their business. You'd never believe it.

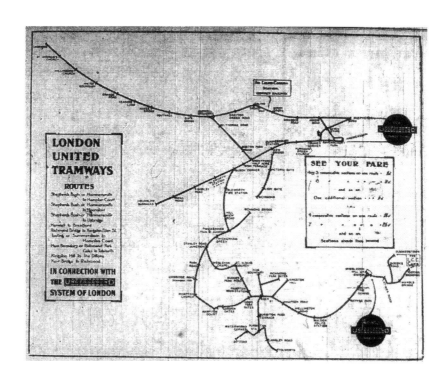

Surrey Comet 1911

Sometimes they gave me a penny for the bus fare, or tuppence, a penny each way, but it was quicker by foot if you went down the Strand. Then I kept the money so that I could buy a tuppenny bar of Nestles chocolate out of the machines. Of course I never had any money over and so whatever money I was given was handy.

I also looked after the stamps. The manager's son was in the office and he would dictate letters to me; little notes that I had to to type and send off. There was Mr Crowley and Mr Foster. They were partners and Mr Foster got twenty pounds a week and I got fifteen bob. He just sat there signing his name; that's all he ever did and they had a typist each. The people I worked with were all pretty decent people though.

After a while he was so interested in these sausage skins that he bought a company out over at Amelia Street at London Bridge and so we all moved over to London Bridge. It was a lousy office though. There was a sort of mirror with metal underneath that reflected the light back into the office; otherwise it would have been like a den.

They had a factory where water was always running along the floor to clean it out and they rolled the sausage skins up and put them into salt water in these barrels.
Sometimes he'd say to me, 'Son, get me a taxi.'
And so I'd run up to the bridge and ride on the running board on the way back.

This was a time when transport was evolving. You had proper taxis now and old fashioned things where the cab was underneath and the driver was sitting above. The horse drawn vehicles were passing out and the motors were coming in.

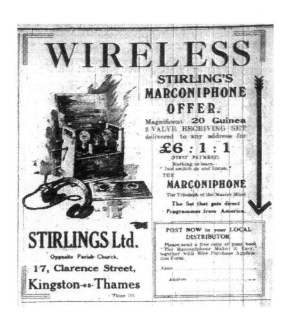

Surrey Comet 1924

CHAPTER 7

Entertainment in the Roaring Twenties!

1920's

ANOTHER CHANGE TO our lives in about 1924 was that the wireless or radio was born. You could make your own set with a cigar box and a crystal and, the only thing was, you had to have earphones and they'd cost you about twenty seven shillings. You could lie in bed and twiddle about with this crystal until you got a signal. There was no charge or anything. Some of my friends had one but I couldn't afford it. It was 27s and 6d for a crystal set with headphones in 1924.

Then they invented sets with valves about the size of an electric light bulb; a big thing burning a lot of heat. You had to tune this in and there was a lot of jiggling about to get a station. Of course there was only London at that time.

The cinemas in those days were the Kinema, The Cinema Palace and The Super Cinema. These were the Flea Pits but then in the late twenties they built a picture palace called the Elite. These were still the silent movies but the cinema was more luxurious.

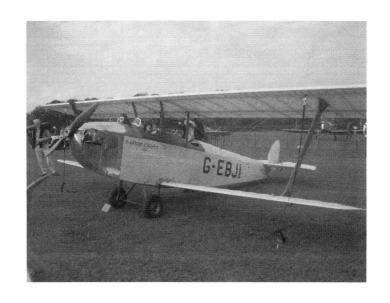

This is a 1924 Hawker Cygnet which still flies
at Old Warden Bedfordshire today.
Norman remembers working on the Hawker Hart Trainer.

3. The Sopwith Aviation Company, which had premises at the old roller rink, Canbury Park Road, Kingston on Thames, first opened in 1915 and had a workforce of over 3,500 people by the end of WW1. After the Great War Tommy Sopwith's bankrupt aviation company's assets were taken over by a group including Harry Hawker, a test pilot. In 1920 HG Hawker Ltd was formed, taking the aircraft, including The Hawker Hind over to Brooklands to fly.

CHAPTER 8

The Hawker's Hurricane
The nuts and bolts of the matter

1925

WHILE I WAS at Cowley on a Sunday night we used to parade in Kingston on The Promenade and all the girls and boys were there. We had a little chat and then moved on. One Sunday it was foggy and I must have been walking on the outside of the path when I put my foot off the curb and my head went through the window of a car. I got such a bump on me head and I've still got a scar today. They did pay me while I was away from work but there was no damage done to my clothes.

Since Mr Clayton was a solicitor my Mother said,

'Can't you do anything?' and so I think he claimed about fifteen pound.

I was sixteen when I left Cowley. After a while my Mother said,

'You can't go on like this. I'm getting nothing out of it.'

My Dad was friendly with his workmate and my Mother used to meet his wife and they kept a sweet shop nearby so my Mother said,

'I'm going over there to get you a job.'

'No you don't,' I said but she didn't take any notice. She was off.

This woman said, 'I'll see my son in law,' and so that's how I got a job at Hawkers3, the aeroplane factory and at first I was in the office, but there was very little for me to do, just a bit of filing and that sort of thing and so I got a bit restless.

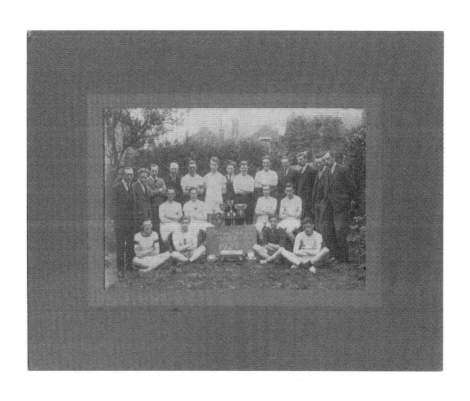

Norman's Athletics Day
Hawkers 1927

I was looking out on to the factory floor one day with all this work going on below and I said to the foreman,

'Can't I go out to work on the floor.'

'Yes, of course you can,' he said.

That's how I started working on the machine shop floor where they produced all the military aircraft like the Hurricane.

I went on a machine called a Capstan Machine and I was a tool setter where I was making little bolts and washers and things like that, in different metals; some were steel, some were brass and some were fibre. I stuck that for a while but then again, I was only getting four pence farthing per hour and so I said to the foreman,

'That bloke in front of me is getting a shilling. Why is that?'

'Well,' he said. 'He's over twenty one.'

So I said, 'So I have to wait until I'm twenty one to get a shilling an hour do I!'

I joined in with the athletics at Hawkers in 1927. I was a 100 yards sprinter and I won! The photo shows the others I worked with at Hawkers. There's the foreman of the machine shop and his son in law. Then there's the fitter, a capstan handler, a charger, a chap on the mills and a labourer, Terry the old man.

We won three cups but I was very ill that day we came home. You see, they'd filled these cups up with beer and wine. Wine was in one and beer was in the other and I mixed them. I didn't know 'til I got home what I'd done and I've never done it since. There you are; my athletic prowess.

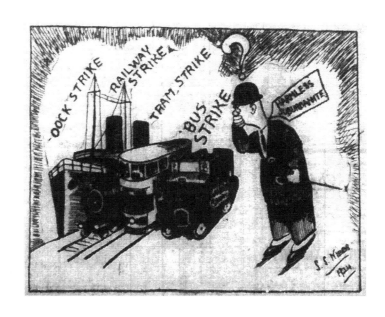

Surrey Comet

CHAPTER 8

400 WOMEN, 200 BOYS WANTED TO SAIL TO AUSTRALIA!
1926

THINGS GOT REALLY hard for people like us at home and my father was out of work more than he was in and then we had the General Strike; it was a very bad period. It affected a lot of people with money and some even committed suicide, but all the other depression was the workers and they lost their jobs.

If that wasn't bad enough, in 1930 we had the big crash, the big Depression, and then we were out of work for a couple of years.

I always I wanted to get away. I wanted to go to Canada or to Australia or get on a boat as a steward. A mate went on the Castle Line to South Africa and when he came home we used to be envious of him.

Another mate of mine said one day,

'I want to get away as well.'

We'd heard that you could apply at one of the shipping offices. There were loads at that time but when we got there we were told that we could only get away if we had fifty pounds for a uniform.

'Where are we going to get fifty pounds from?' I said.

Then we heard that the New Zealand Shipping Company would take people on at the port, so we got up early one morning and went down to the docks and we found this ship.

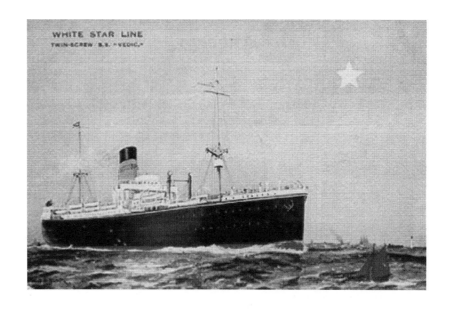

The Vedic
White Star Line

This mate of mine looked at me and I looked at him and we got a bit nervous and so we turned away. Then, as we were coming down Victoria Street to the bottom near Blackfriars, we saw this big banner:

'400 WOMEN, 200 BOYS WANTED TO SAIL TO AUSTRALIA.'

We went straight in. No hesitation. That's how it happened. We went in there and this man said,

'Well, yes, we want you. Report to the officer at the Salvation Army in Kingston to see if you are eligible.'

Unfortunately I wasn't because I was only seventeen at the time and you had to be eighteen but we were given all the information, the name of the ship, the name of the captain and when the boat was going to sail and I was so excited to go that I went back and said,

'By the time that ship sails on 15th October I shall be eighteen.'

'Oh, OK then,' the man said and that's how I got in. They asked me nothing else.

I didn't need a medical or anything; they just needed labour in Australia.

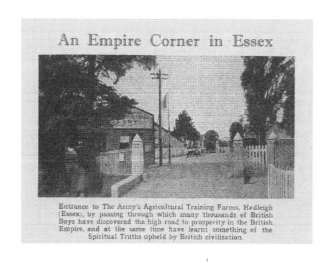

An Empire Corner in Essex

Entrance to The Army's Agricultural Training Farms, Hadleigh (Essex), by passing through which many thousands of British Boys have discovered the high road to prosperity in the British Empire, and at the same time have learnt something of the Spiritual Truths upheld by British civilization.

6. During the 1920's families and farm boys were given assisted passages to a new life in Australia by the Salvation Army. They chartered vessels including The Vedic, which transported immigrants four times in the late 1920's. Over 400 young men a year were trained at a farm colony set up by William Booth at Hadleigh in Essex before departure.

CHAPTER 9

Apple picking!

Summer 1927

I REMEMBER WHEN I came home to tell my Mother my plans and showed her the photo of the ship and I said to her,

'This is the ship I'm going to travel to Australia on. *The Vedic.*'

'We'll see about that,' she replied. 'Wait 'til your Father comes home.'

But when he came home I was so surprised because he agreed with me. Of course he was a bit of a wanderer himself when he was younger. He went up to Newcastle and to Barrow in Furness to work up in the north of England. He was cheeky like I was, so I suppose the travel bug was in him too, so that was that.

Just before I went to Australia I hadn't seen much of Mae because she was in and out of service but, do you know what, she was always there! She was there in the background. It didn't matter where she was, but she was there.

Then we heard from the Salvation Army and they said that we had to go to their farm, Hadleigh Farm in Essex6 for six weeks. It was comical. They called it farm training.

We were down there for six weeks and it was fruit harvesting, plums and apples, and that was all the training, picking fruit. It was all cheap labour, I mean, when you got to Australia what did you get, £1 a week! It was all cheap labour.

We picked fruit and I weighed in at 9 stone 6 and I came out at 10 stone 6. So they fed us well. We had big meals at lunchtime but we were also eating this fruit all the morning, so we were really filling ourselves up.

A Pioneer in Empire Migration and Settlement

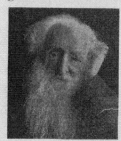

The Founder of The Salvation Army

who was in Christchurch, New Zealand, when the S.S. *Vancouver*, the first ship to sail under The Army Flag, left Liverpool for Canada, on 26th April, 1905. The message he dispatched to passengers then proceeding to Canada is not inappropriate to-day to migrants proceeding on the S.S. *Vedic* to Australia :

'GOD carry you safely to your new home. Fearlessly calculate upon hard work. Bravely meet difficulties. Do your duty by your families. Help your comrades. Make a home overseas that will be a credit to the Old Land. Put God first. Stand by The Army. Save your souls. Meet me in Heaven.'

24th April, 1905.   *WILLIAM BOOTH.*

Page Two

William Booth
Pioneer in Migration

Do you know what? There seemed to be a very queer thing in our favour. Every Saturday morning it rained, so we didn't do any work; we just went in the barn. It cleared up in the afternoon so off we went to Southend for the rest of the day. I'll always remember we were sitting there and the boys were singing and the rain came down and the boys would say,

'Send it down David, send it down.'

So afterwards we went down to Southend to have a bit of fun.

We weren't allowed to smoke but we were all smokers in those days, but there was an area in the farm where there was a slope and we used to hide down there to have a smoke. There was also a gangway leading to the farm and there was this little shop, a sort of cafe, and we sat in there to smoke too.

We walked to the station, which was a couple of stations away from Southend and I remember one day I was smoking and I when looked down my pocket was all alight. Some live ash had dropped down and burnt a hole in my pocket!

Of course we used to sleep about thirty in the dormitory and there was a bit of a show at night time, as you can imagine, getting us all bedded down.

Another thing I remember is that the Salvation Army is an Army. You've got the soldiers, the sergeants, the lieutenants and you've got the Captain in charge all up to General Booth, as he was then. It was all run like an army. The Major was in charge of the camp and I remember that it was our last day so we all decided we'd go over to the barbers to have a shave.

He walked in, 'Shame,' he barked. 'You won't be able to do this when you go to Australia you know.'

So he didn't approve of that.

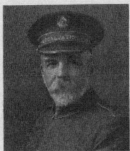

COMMISSIONER DAVID C. LAMB.
Director of The Salvation Army Migration and
Settlement Department

My DEAR FRIEND,

You are favoured to be on the *Vedic*, since thousands applied who desired to sail to Australia under The Army Flag. I hope you will have a pleasant, comfortable, and happy voyage. You will, no doubt, be at once confronted with some disappointments and difficulties : the accommodation on the ship will, perhaps, be different to what you expect : your cabin companions may not be such as you would have chosen, yet it may be all just the reverse ! Much will depend upon your willingness and ability to adapt yourself to strange conditions at the commencement of a new life.

Farewell Message

CHAPTER 10

Saying Farewell to England

October 1927

BACK AT HOME we had a big party when we were about to leave. My mate and his family lived down the road, so they all came up to the party and other members of the street came in too. We were indoors and all over the place because you couldn't get everyone inside.

Mae was away in service at that time and so she didn't come to the party. We were now 18 and couldn't see much of each other.

Then we went to the Guildhall in London where we met the Lord Mayor, the Captain of the ship and there were some other dignitaries there as well, from high up in the Salvation Army. We had a sort of service to wish us well. To be honest with you we were too excited to get on this ship to take much notice of that night.

Then we went straight up to Liverpool on the night train.

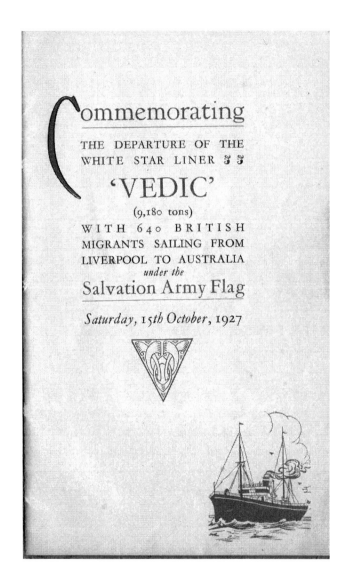

Commemorating

THE DEPARTURE OF THE
WHITE STAR LINER S S

'VEDIC'

(9,180 tons)

WITH 640 BRITISH
MIGRANTS SAILING FROM
LIVERPOOL TO AUSTRALIA
under the

Salvation Army Flag

Saturday, 15th October, 1927

CHAPTER 11

All Aboard who's going Aboard!

Saturday 15th October 1927

WE GOT UP to Liverpool in the morning at about six o'clock. I know we did look around at the shops because I remember buying a razor, a Wardonia Razor. The Gillette was all metal but the underside of this one was sort of fibre, ebonite or something like that. There was more space between the blade and the back which gave you an easier shave.

At about ten in the morning we went aboard the ship. We had to go out by boat because *The Vedic* was moored in the river. We sailed on 15th October 1927.

On deck they said, 'In three days time you'll be in nice warm weather.'

And we were, in three days time we were off the coast of Portugal.

I must have taken a case or something but I just don't remember. I do remember that I took an overcoat, with a velvet collar. It'd been nicked I think. My Dad used to be friends with a chap up in Hook and he used to be a bookie's runner. In the local race meetings at Epsom and Ascot he'd have a marquee and ran a pub. He had an old bloke helping him who stopped in there at night and guarded the place, because the burglars used to come in, so they had to bury the cash in the ground each night and there'd often be someone creeping in trying to find it. Old George there, he'd bang them on the hand and they'd go off crying.

He was a bit of a roamer Old George my Dad's friend; he used to roam about all over the country, but he was always there at these meetings, and he used to go around cars nicking things, mostly overcoats.

So I remember my Dad gave me this overcoat with a nice velvet collar; a beautiful coat; must have been worth a lot of money. So I took it with me to Australia.

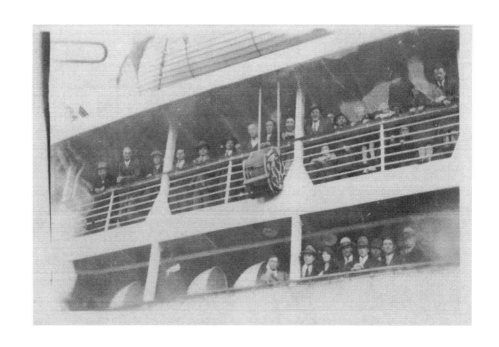

On the Vedic

It must have been in the afternoon when we sailed because, as we went down the coast it got darker, and by Cornwall it was pitch black. We stayed on deck until there was nothing to see and then we went below. I know the *The Vedic* had been an old cargo ship that was converted into a passenger ship and it was only 9,000 tonnes.

The Bay of Biscay was not too bad, but sometimes you'd get the pitch and toss and sometimes you'd get a roll, so you'd go inside and one moment you'd see the sky through the port hole but the next moment you'd see the water.

After four days a bloke said,
    'If you get up now you'll see The Canary Islands on the right hand side, and that was when we saw the flying fish too!

Another couple of days and we were off the coast of Africa and it was, phew, so hot. There was no air. The sea was as calm as a mill pond; not a ripple; only what the ship made and so we got down there to Cape Town on 5th November. Three weeks.

I don't know whether I told you before but that's when they brought the locals down with the coal and each had a basket on their shoulder which they would fill up with coal, bring it down, tip it and come up the other side. They were chanting all night as they worked. We stayed there two nights while they loaded us up but we all stayed on board.

We had six bunks in the cabin, but in the day time we were up on deck. We had no jobs to do because we were passengers. We'd paid ten pound for that. That was the first job as soon as you got to Australia, to pay it back. They took half your wages, 10 shillings a week. On the ship up at the other end there were four baths and six for washing. In hot weather we used to lay in the salt water bath to keep cool.

General Booth's Message to You !

YOU are going over the sea, with its possible storms, to a Country with its unknown difficulties, in order to find conditions more favourable to your earthly welfare than those you at present enjoy.

I wish you every blessing and assure you that with industry, truthfulness, honesty, and the Service of God you have good ground for expecting a welcome success.

On the other side of the Sea of Life there is a land of pure delight, where poverty, sickness, and death never come, and I want every one of you to meet me on those eternal shores.

The Salvation Ship bound for that celestial Country is ready to sail. Jesus Christ has bought you a free passage. If you have not started, enter your name forthwith, bid farewell to every evil way, hurry on board and sail with us, not only to your new home but to Eternal Glory.

Your true friend and General,

Bramwell Booth.

International Headquarters,
London, E.C.

I don't think we were all that interested in women. We were going to a new life, but they must have stowed the girls somewhere else because they seemed to come out of the woodwork when we arrived. We hardly saw any of them until the end.

I had a ring on my finger and kept forgetting it. The first time I went back to my bunk to look for it and it was still there, but on another day I never noticed it missing at first, but I then went, 'Oh!' (looking at my hand), and it was gone.

The ring was from a cousin of mine, my second cousin. My dad's first cousin. She was adopted by my grandmother; one of six children. She never married and she was part of the family, more like a sister to my father. All the children thought the world of her.

The worst night was in the Indian Ocean. I was asleep and we were getting battered all over the place. BANG and BANG. I thought, how are we going to get through this? We were smashing about all over the place. That was two or three nights before we got to Australia.

A Few Don'ts

Don't be easily discouraged.

Don't spend your money carelessly.

Don't be afraid of honest work of any kind.

Don't lend money to your fellow-passengers.

Don't gamble. You will need all your money.

Don't listen to persons who offer to change notes.

Don't magnify the drawbacks and ignore the advantages overseas.

Don't fail to report yourself to the nearest Corps, if you are a Salvationist.

Don't tell the Australians how to do their work; they have their own methods.

Don't confide your private affairs to any one you did not know before you sailed.

Don't trust strangers, and be careful about entering into money transactions with them.

Don't forget when desiring to make arrangements for the migration of your friends that The Army's Organization is world-wide.

Don't forget that you can nominate friends in the Homeland and thus make it easy for them to join you in Australia; but nominate through our Organization.

Don't think you are likely to take some one else's job, nor that every newcomer is a competitor for your job. In a well-ordered state every honest worker produces more than he consumes, and the commonwealth is enriched thereby.

Don't scandalize.

> Tell tale tit,
> Your tongue shall be slit,
> And all the sharks in the sea
> Shall have a little bit!

Australian Words, Phrases, and Expressions

ABO.—An abbreviation of the word aboriginal (a native black) frequently used in Australian journalism.

ANTIPODES.—A term which signifies places on the earth's surface directly opposite to each other. Hence its frequent application to Australia by English writers.

AUSSIE.—An abbreviation of the word Australian, now almost universally used by outsiders in a familiar sense to denote an Australian citizen.

BAAL.—An aboriginal word expressing dislike, frequently used in the wording of humorous jokes concerning blacks.

BACK OF BEYOND.—A picturesque allusion to the interior regions of Australia.

BACK-BLOCKS.—The inland settlement areas and townships.

BAIL.—A wooden frame designed to secure a cow's head while being milked.

BANANALANDER.—A term used in certain southern journals to denote a Queenslander.

BANDICOOT.—A bush animal, about the size of a rabbit, which prowls about at night-time in search of roots and insects.

BANG-TAIL MUSTER.—A muster of cattle in which the hairy end of each one's tail is cut off to show it has been counted.

BATHURST BURR.—A spiny, bean-shaped pod which grows on a weed and is notorious for attaching itself to the wool of passing sheep.

BILLABONG.—A small offshoot from a river which rejoins it in wet seasons at a lower point.

BILLY.—A tin container with a wire handle attached used for domestic purposes and, invariably, in the bush for carrying and boiling water. A billy-can.

BILLY TEA.—Tea made in the open by using a billy-can.

BLACK-BIRDING.—The act of kidnapping South Sea Islanders from their island homes which became common during the time when they were universally employed on Queensland sugar plantations.

BLACK-BUTT.—A common species of the gum-tree or Eucalyptus possessing a black base.

BLACKTRACKER.—An aboriginal expert in tracking people through the bush by detecting their trail.

BLUE-GUM.—A common species of the Eucalyptus. Generally pronounced 'Blueg'm.'

BLUEY.—A swagman's blanket, blue being recognized as the most favoured colour.

BOARD.—The portion of the floor of the shearing shed on which the sheep are shorn.

BONZER.—A very common slang word denoting satisfaction. Good. A corruption of 'bonanza.'

BOOMERANG.—A curved piece of wood used for hunting and as a weapon of war by the black tribes.

BORONIA.—A sweet-scented, bush wildflower, of which there are several species.

BOSKER.—A slang word used as an adjective to denote good quality or appreciation.

BOSS-COCKIE.—A small farmer who works himself, but also employs labour.

BOUNDARY RIDER.—A man employed continually to inspect the boundary fences of a station.

BOWYANGS.—Knee bands of rope or leather used by labourers.

BRAMBLE.—Dried bush leaves used in the kindling of a fire.

BRUMBY.—A wild horse. The derivation of the word is indefinite.

BRUSH-TURKEY.—A native bird resembling the domestic hen turkey, but smaller in size. It builds its nest in the shape of a huge mound in which several lay their eggs.

A Few Do's and Don'ts

74

In sight of Australia at last

We didn't have any more stops after that, only Albany in Western Australia and I think it was mostly girls that disembarked at that one before we set off again.

Then it was another week's sail to Melbourne. Everything was new to us. You were going to a land six weeks away before you could get in touch with anybody. We came into dock at the River Yarrow and I got off with all the boys at Melbourne.

On the very last night this girl was talking to me and it was as if she'd known me all my life but it was such a shame because she was going to get off in the morning. We were up on the deck chatting away and it was a lovely evening but all I could think of was that I wouldn't see her again.

On the same day there was a bloke with a desk on deck and we lined up to go up to him and he would size you up and tell you where you were going to be sent. Then, the next morning we got off the boat and were packed on to a train and were taken to our destination.

Everything was exciting. We were going to get a new job, a new outlook, new everything!

SILKY OAK.—A tree which produces a high grade furniture wood. It is plentiful in Queensland.

SLAB.—A heavy, roughly-cut plank.

SLIP-RAIL.—A fence rail made to be removable and serve as a gateway.

SOUTH AUSTRALIA.—The central southern State of Australia.

SOUTHERLY BUSTER.—A strong, gusty wind peculiar to a section of the East Coast of New South Wales.

SOUTHERN CROSS.—A constellation, visible in all parts of the Southern Hemisphere and accepted as the emblem of Australia.

SPRUIKER.—A slang word denoting a platform speaker.

SPRINGER.—A cow approaching milking period.

SQUIRT.—The slang word for revolver.

SQUATTER.—A large sheep or cattle run owner. A pastoralist.

STAGHORN.—A beautiful bush growth which resembles its name.

STATION.—A cattle or sheep run, the property of a squatter or pastoralist.

STICKY-BEAK.—A slang term denoting an inquisitive person.

STINGAREE.—A flat-bodied sea inhabitant, half reptile, half fish, capable of inflicting a painful sting with its tail.

STOCK-HORSE.—A horse trained to muster and draft cattle.

STOCKMAN.—A man in charge of the cattle on a run.

STOCK-RIDER.—A man who spends his time on horseback guarding cattle on unfenced areas.

STOCK-ROUTE.—A route permitted by law across station property for the use of travelling stock.

STOCK-WHIP.—A long greenhide whip used by stockmen.

STORE CATTLE.—Cattle in the course of being fattened for sale.

STRINGY-BARK.—A species of gum possessing a tough fibrous bark removable in sheets and often used in roofing bush huts.

SULKY.—A light two-wheeled vehicle drawn by one horse, also styled a trap.

SUNDOWNER.—An outback swagman, so-called as he is said to make sundown the hour of his arrival at a homestead. The word is now almost obsolete, swaggie being the term almost universally in use.

SWAG.—A swagman's bundle, containing tent, blanket, etc.

SWAGGIE.—A nomad who, carrying a swag, tramps from place to place. A swagman.

TAKE-DOWN.—A slang word for thief. A cheat.

TASMANIA.—The island State of the Commonwealth.

TASMANIAN DEVIL.—A nocturnal, browsing animal.

TASMANIAN TIGER.—An animal of the hyena type being fast exterminated.

TASSY.—A familiar way of alluding to Tasmania. The pronunciation is Tazzy.

TEA TREE.—A shrub from the leaves of which a tea can be made.

THONG.—The leather body of a whip.

THROWING-STICK.—An aboriginal weapon with which spears are hurled.

TIGER CAT.—A powerful night prowling animal, destructive to poultry and resembling in appearance a huge cat.

TIPSLINGER.—The slang term for racecourse tipster.

TO 'BACK AND FILL.'—To avoid the point at issue.

TO BE A 'FAIR COW.'—To be excessively disagreeable.

TO BE A 'FINANCIAL' MEMBER.—To have paid one's due subscription

TO BE A 'PUT-UP JOB.'—To be previously arranged.

TO BE 'BUSHED.'—To be lost, to be non-plussed.

TO BE 'ON THE OUTER.'—To be penniless.

TO BE 'ON THE TRACK.'—To be tramping from place to place.

TO BE 'ON THE WALLABY.'—As above.

TO BE 'ROUGH AS BAGS.'—To be uncouth.

TO BE 'THE PURE MERINO.'—To show good breeding.

TO BE 'UP TO PUTTY.'—To be no good.

TO 'BOTTOM ON TO GOLD.'—To strike gold. To succeed.

Norman wanted to be
'The Pure Merine' and not
'Up to Putty!'

CHAPTER 12

Norman Down Under!

End of November 1927

WHEN WE GOT to Australia it was terribly hot and these blokes came aboard to do the unloading and one of them said,

'You're not going to need that overcoat mate. It's like this all the time.'

Of course I didn't need anything on at all actually because the heat was getting to me, so I said, 'There you are.'

I must have had a case or something too, but when you got on the boat you had to go down the hole and so I didn't see anything so what I left with I don't know; just what I stood up in I suppose.

I was put on one of the jobs the farthest away and so it was going to be quite a journey, but I couldn't get there in a day so I had to stop overnight. I didn't have much money on me so they gave me 2 shillings for bed, 2 shillings for a light meal and 2 shillings for a breakfast.

I got off at this station called The Rock and I was supposed to go on the following morning to a place called Lockhart, which was my final destination. I was on the station and there were carriages on a siding by the side of the track and, since I'm always one for making money I thought, well, I could sleep on this bench on the station or I could sleep in one of those carriages so I dossed down in there for the night and saved myself two bob.

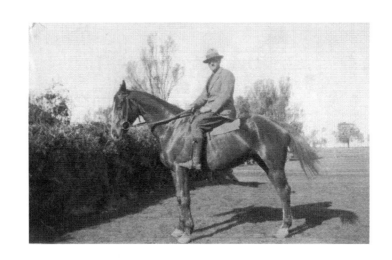

Norman Learns to ride in
New South Wales

My friend was sent up to North West Victoria to a dairy farm. His name was Fred Smith. I never saw him for quite a while as I went to New South Wales which was where I started.

I must have thought about Mae when I went to Australia because I sent her a snapshot. We must have corresponded for a while. I know I wrote to her in the early days but it dropped off. The only thing I promised was that I'd write to my Mother every week, because if you only wrote now and again it'd be weeks before you'd get an answer. If you wrote once a week then hopefully you'd get a reply back every week. It took six weeks to get over and six weeks to get back. That's three months before you got an answer. That was that.

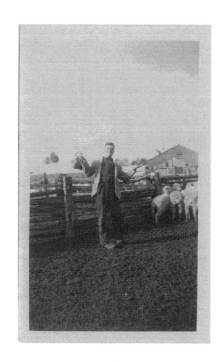

Easy!

I was taken on by a woman farm owner but she had a manager working for her and he was an ex army man. I think he was her boyfriend. Anyway, he wasn't too bad a bloke; a bit difficult at times but I was a devil for lying in bed. I had an alarm clock but I often slept right through it.

So he said, 'Put it in a kerosene tin and see how that works.'

So that made more noise and that woke me up. One time though I was still asleep and he chucked a jug of water over me. Cor Blimey, I never slept after that.

He said,' You gotta get up!'

Anyway this didn't help matters. There were two other English boys who worked on the farm further over and they used to come over to the one I was on.

Besides me, the manager had an Irishman and he used to do all the harvesting with the wheat side of the business and I looked after the sheep but I also did the milking and general jobs around the house too. I moved the sheep from one paddock to another on horseback or when the fences broke I mended them. You never went anywhere without a horse. There weren't many motors about at that time but the farmer had one.

Once it came on to harvest time these English blokes used to get me going and say,

'You wanna tell them that you were up until 11 o'clock working last night.'

So I wrote a letter to the Salvation Army and the farm manager got a stinking letter back. That didn't help matters between us because they weren't allowed to keep me up so late after that.

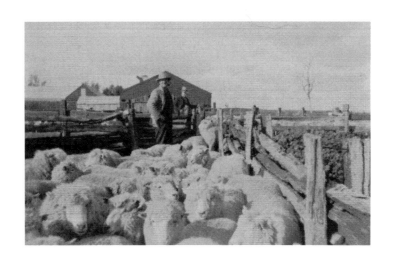

Norman, the shepherd

I used to see a bloke down the road going by, taking the wheat up to the siding, and I got chatting to him one day and he said,

'Yes, I'll take you on.'

So I transferred to him but he was a real Tartar.

When the Australians came back from the war they were allotted 640 acres and some managed it and some didn't, but he did. He built himself a brick house and he bought his mate's blocks too, because they didn't get on with them, so he got two or three big blocks.

I was helping him out with the wheat and with the sheep and milking and then his wife used to go away to her people for a month for a holiday and he said,

'Mate, you're the chief cook now too.'

And so I'd do the cooking and they'd come in and I'd give them something. I did find out how to make Junket and they said,

'Don't you know how to make anything else besides Junket?'

'No' I said and laughed. 'It's so easy to do.'

I remember the fruit trees out there. There were apricots, nectarines and peaches and so we had a lot of fresh fruit. We also had corned beef and potatoes.

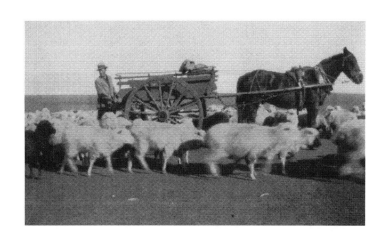

Norman at work

Easter 1928

I was in bed one day and it was Easter and he said,

'Get up!'

But I said, 'It's holiday.'

'Holiday!' he said. 'No holidays at Easter. Get out there. The animals have got to be fed.'

I said, 'We always have a holiday at Easter.'

He said 'You'll die in that bed.'

I said, 'I won't. I'm off!'

So I finished up with him and got back with the other bloke I first started with. That carried on for a while but he had a mate staying with him who'd broken his arm.

The owner said, 'You take on the wheat.'

A couple of days later his father died and he said,

'I gotta go.'

So the owner said to me,

'You'll have to do it.'

I said, 'If I have to do it then I want to get what you were paying him.'

'Oh no,' he said.

I said, 'If I have to do it then I want what he got paid.'

'Oh no!' he said.

So I said, 'I'm off!'

He said, 'You can't do that. You're a quitter.'

'Whatever, I'm off,' I said and that was that, so I left him to do it himself.

I don't know what happened. I was a bit of a lad really but I didn't like being treated unfairly, so I was twelve months up there but then I went down to what they used to call the Big Smoke.

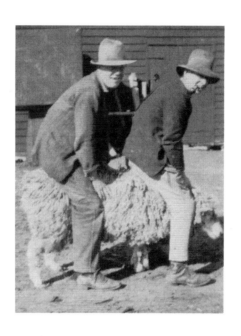

Ready to Sheer the Sheep!

There was a place, down there in Melbourne, not like a hotel but it was rooms called Excells. There was an agency underneath so you'd have a room above, but you'd also have the first choice looking round at the jobs in the morning before he opened, so we always used to stop there. That's where I met up with Fred Smith for the first time since arriving in Australia.

I remember there were two and sometimes three beds in a room but mine was a two bed this time. Anyway, I met old Fred and he came into our room and he sneaked in and up the stairs but soon it was getting late. It was midnight and we were still laughing.

Someone shouted. 'Shurrup, we want to get some sleep.'
So we had to quieten down.
'What are we going to do with him?' I said.
We couldn't get him out so he had to stay there all night and he slept on the floor so that was the first time I met up with old Fred again.

Then I got this job up at Wycheproof. That was just for wheat carting and I went up there for six weeks. There was a farm opposite and he was a Scotch man. It was Christmas time and he said,
'Would you like to come over and have Christmas lunch with us?'

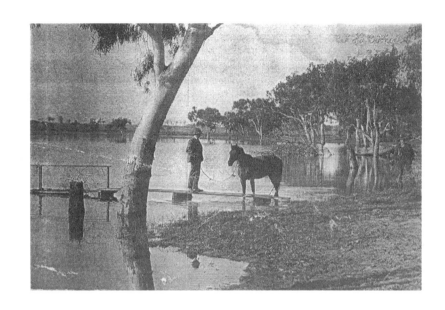

Brown's Lake

Christmas 1928

So we went over to his place and had a Christmas lunch but we came back to splash in the water. I must explain here that there was a hill and they dug a trench and the water came down into this water hole for the animals to feed and they called it a dam. The water in the dam looked dirty; muddy really, and so when we came out from lunch in the afternoon we went for a splash in this dam. I remember that because there were crayfish in the water biting our toes. How the devil did they get crayfish in there?

There were others in the family, boys and girls, and they used to come and meet somehow. Sometimes they said,
> 'We're gonna into town to a wine bar, would you like to join us?'
> 'Yer ok,' we said and so off we went to the wine bar.

So, I enjoyed my time in Wycheproof but after that he said,
> 'I'm afraid I can't keep you on, because I can't afford it.'

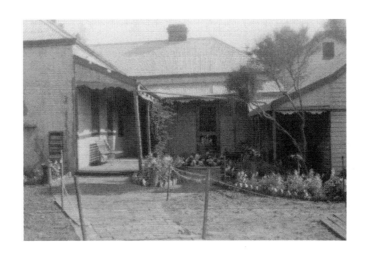

Kimbolton Station

So then I went back to the Big Smoke and I got talking to a bloke who said, 'I'm taking on a big block down on the south coast at a place called Timboon, near Port Campbell. There's a man down there who wants someone to help him. Would you like to come?'

This bloke had a horse and a gig and he was going to Timboon to start his block off.   Let me explain; he'd been allocated a square mile of land, 640 acres, and that was called a block. He was going to clear it to start a farm, so I went down with him. Half way down he just hobbled his horse and then it couldn't go anywhere, just feed around.

Hobbled is when you tie the front legs together like handcuffs. After that you put a tarpaulin over the shafts and then we could sit under there to kip for the night. It was just the one night and the next day we arrived at Timboon.

I didn't stay there very long either. He wanted me to take a block on by myself but I couldn't stay. There were blocks and they'd cleared thirty acres and tried to make a living but they hadn't cleared anymore. I knew that if you did take a block on, then you'd have to clear so much before the government gave you a grant to get an animal and a shelter. You made a start and then they supported you for a bit until you'd cleared the whole thing and you could make a good living out of it. I thought, that'll be a long job, so it wasn't for me.

I had six weeks of helping him. We cut all the shorter stuff down but there were a lot of trees. He gave me some dynamite and we were blowing up trees, clearing the scrub.

One day he said, 'Oh Norman, I'm sorry but I'm afraid I can't afford to pay you.'

'OK,' I said and so it was back to town looking for work again.

I used to write to my mother every week. I put the address on the top and when I moved on they'd send the post on to me. That's the way we kept in touch.

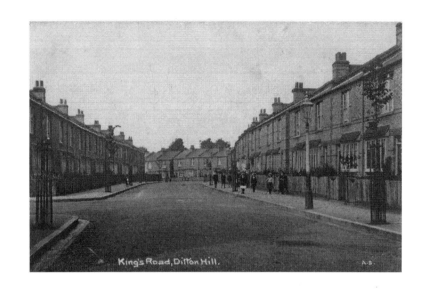

Kings Road Ditton Hill

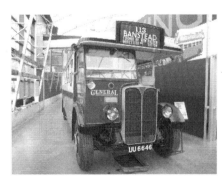

The Kingston to Sutton bus 1929
The 113
in the Brooklands Museum

CHAPTER 13

News from England

1929

WHILE I WAS away The Halifax Building Society people came along to my mum and dad's.

He said, 'We've bought these houses and we can give you fifty pounds to get out or we'll get a financial advisor round and you can buy them back for £275.'

So then they had these options. Tough really. Well, the rent at that time was thirteen and a penny; including rates.

The advisor came round and said,

'This is what it works out to. Thirteen shillings a week and you've got thirty years to pay it in.'

So it turned out less than the rent. Buying a house on the dole! I mean, it seemed to be stupid, but it was forced on people. They were buying the house for what you paid in rent. The only thing was, you had to have a twenty five pound deposit.

Where were they going to get twenty five pound from? I think they had about twelve pounds saved and so my dad jumped on his bike and went down to see his sister in Kent and her husband was an engine driver on the railway, so he had a regular job. They were wealthy people and never used to squander money, so they used to save. Dad borrowed twelve or fourteen pounds off my aunt to make up the twenty five pounds. So that's how they got started.

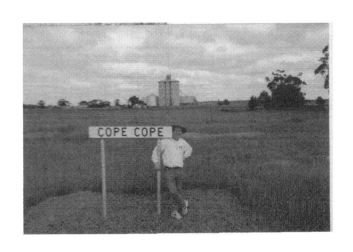

All there is left of Cope Cope today!

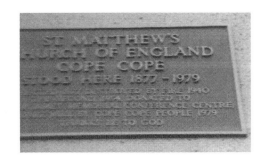

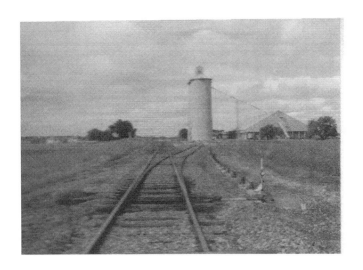

CHAPTER 14

Back in Australia

Winter 1929

WELL, THIS TIME back in the Big Smoke I saw this job up at Cope Cope and I applied for it and stayed there for two and a half years. I dealt with the sheep, did the milking and made the butter. The milk used to separate and then you had the cream. Then you left the cream until the end of the week and made that into butter. That was part of my job.

There was a drought all the time I was there. There was quite a big lake but when the drought broke, the lake filled up in two days and overflowed into two salt lakes. That was brackish water, as clear as a bell but you couldn't drink it, whereas they had what they called the Dam, which was a muddy looking pond, but drinkable.

There were two farms altogether. Part of it was down to wheat and the other part to sheep. The farmer Mr Brown owned all the property. Mr Stewart was a share cropper. He supplied all the horses and the machinery but the man that owned the farm, he got half of the crop and so he was on to a good thing. All he did was let them grow on his land and he reaped half of the profit. He brought up his family on that.

When we were there we went into Donald sometimes to have a few beers. When I was at Cope Cope it was a dying town. We didn't know that at the time, but it had this big lake and I think once they had three pubs and four hotels there. It was a thriving place because when the railways came it finished at Cope Cope and that's where the town rose from. When I arrived there 100 years later it had descended and many of the pubs had gone, but today all that's left is that sign, Cope Cope; nothing else. The railway went on and they developed Donald which became the main town.

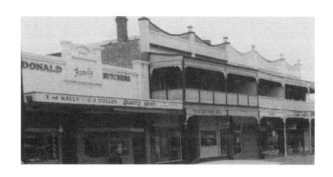

Donald, little changed today

While I was in Australia there were no pictures in Cope Cope but then I found out that they had a big garage in Donald and sometimes they would put a film on there but even that was eight miles away. At the same time down at The Big Smoke things were all happening.

'We are going to have Talkies,' they said.

At first it was fifty percent Talkies and then it was full Talkies. So, when I had any spare time I used to go down to Melbourne and sometimes I went to the pictures three times in the one day!

I'd been in Australia for four years when my mum asked me to come home to help. It took six months to pay off the Salvation Army because I only had a pound a week in wages. I couldn't send anything home out of a pound! With the rate of exchange that'd only be fourteen bob.

At the same time Fred wrote as well because he wanted to go back too. His folks had also written to him and so it was agreed between us to go back home. I don't really remember how I did it but then I had to start to save up for the fare.

Well Fred, he was a bit of a dare devil. A lot of them used to go riding on the sides of the freight trains like they do in America. They'd jump off just as the train pulled into the next station. Fred had travelled to New South Wales and he got in with the people there and played football and all sorts with them, but he hurt his knee playing football. Once he was jumping off this train as it was coming into the station and his knee gave way. He lay down but, from what I gather, he raised his head up and the train caught him just like that. Smack. That was it. So that was the end of poor old Fred. He was always a dare devil. I remember when we were up in the fields near here in Ditton when we were young and we'd dare him to get on a horse. He'd always have a go would Fred.

People took care of him over there and sent the ashes back to his mother and father and they had it printed in the paper, which they sent on back to me. Fred died a year before I came home, but I didn't know over there. It took six weeks for the news to come back to England and another six weeks for it to get back to Australia, so it was four or five months before I knew about it. And I was there.

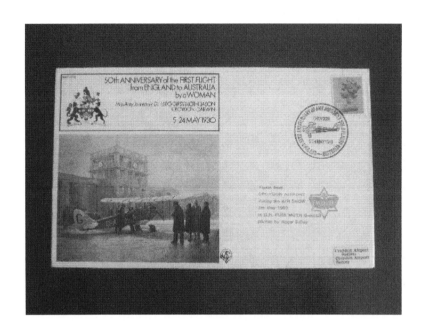

First Day Cover Celebrating
Trail Blazers!

Other Trail Blazers of their Time

1930

In the papers I read the news of Amy Johnson. At that time she landed in the north of Australia, far away from where I was. She picked up with Morrison and so she drifted around Australia with him, I think, and then they got married and came back here and next they blazed a trail to South Africa.

I don't think Amy Johnson was very rich and so I thought, she's another person like me, out exploring the world. I admired her though. What she did was amazing.

1937

Then there was Amelia Earhart. She got to Australia too. That was after I'd come home, but I was excited to hear of her progress with excitement. After all, I was proud that I'd been there too.

Do you know, all those years ago women were trail blazers in flying? It must have been a wonderful time. It wasn't until the 50's and 60's that women got emancipated wasn't it? It was even the late 20's before they got to vote!

It just proved to me that it wasn't just the rich and famous who did these things.

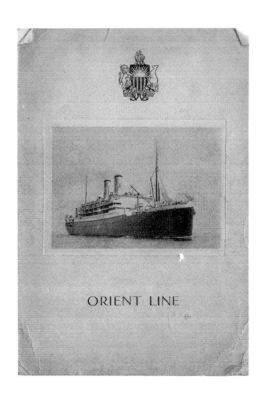

The SS Orama

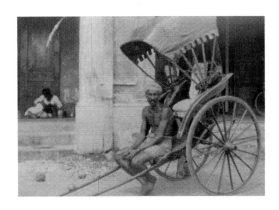

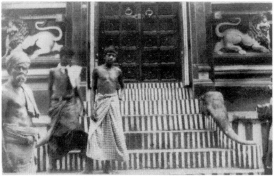

Ceylon (Sri Lanka)

CHAPTER 16

Finding my Way Back Home

July 1931

ON THE JOURNEY home we left Port Melbourne sailing on the *SS Orama* on The Orient Line. We had a rough trip though the Great Australian Bight, the sea between Melbourne and Freemantle. It should have taken up six days but it took us eight days and everyone was sea sick.

I said to one of the crew,

'How on earth do you lose two days? You run these boats on time. You say you're gonna sail on a certain day months ahead in the paper. You say, this boat will depart from Melbourne on 24th July 1931, yet you've lost two days just coming across the Bight.'

'Oh,' he said. 'We can make that up. The only place we may not make it on times is at the mouth of the Thames. That's the only place we can get caught. They drop the mail off at Plymouth so that it reaches London before the ship gets to the Thames though. You'll see.'

It was very stormy until we got to Freemantle. It was strange because when you walk on the boat you get your sea legs, but when you get off again you put your feet on the stairs to go down to the toilet say, but you keep wanting the floor to go down, but it doesn't. It was funny trying to get your land legs again. You get sea legs and land legs.

Then we went on to Colombo. We didn't dock there because it wasn't deep enough, but we did go ashore by boat. I think we were only there one day, but when you anchor all these people come on board in these gowns, that's their local clothes, wanting you to go to their hotel to have a meal.

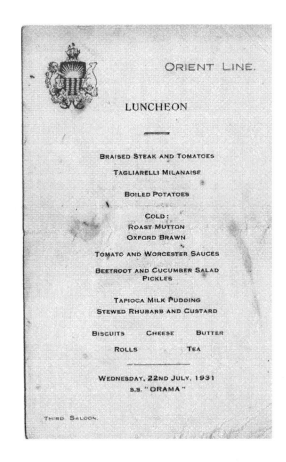

ORIENT LINE.

LUCHEON

BRAISED STEAK AND TOMATOES

TAGLIARELLI MILANAISE

BOILED POTATOES

COLD:
ROAST MUTTON
OXFORD BRAWN

TOMATO AND WORCESTER SAUCES

BEETROOT AND CUCUMBER SALAD
PICKLES

TAPIOCA MILK PUDDING
STEWED RHUBARB AND CUSTARD

BISCUITS   CHEESE   BUTTER

ROLLS   TEA

WEDNESDAY, 22ND JULY, 1931
S.S. "ORAMA"

THIRD SALOON.

Also you get conjurers coming on deck, Indians who produce live chicks before your eyes! How the hell do they do that? They're sitting down on the deck and they produce these chicks. Unbelievable! There were snake charmers too. All that sort of thing.

I made friends with three fellas and one girl and we used to sit on one part of the deck every day having our breakfast together and having a chin wag, so when we did go ashore we kept in a group together. Frank was the name of one of the friends. Janet was one of the girls, a Scotch girl. Then there was a boy from Newcastle. There were just the four of us. Every day we used to sit on the deck and chat and other times of the day you'd be on your own and looking over the side of the boat watching all the water go by. You'd just sit like that for ages.

There was one woman who came aboard on a stretcher because she was sea sick before she came on. Strange that. Auto suggestion you know. She only had to touch a boat and she was sick. She never saw a thing while she was on board and then she went off on the stretcher too!

The dining room was the whole width of the ship and I've got lots of the menus. Coming back the passengers were all mixed, men and women together. You'd talk and in the evening you'd lean on the bench and watch the water. Hours you'd watch the water.

We didn't play cards or do any reading. We might have played some deck games, quoits and things like that. There was a swimming bath but I don't remember going in it. I don't remember doing any washing. Did I live in what I had on and that was that? Must have been. The crew never had any time to do anything either. They were always on the go all the time.

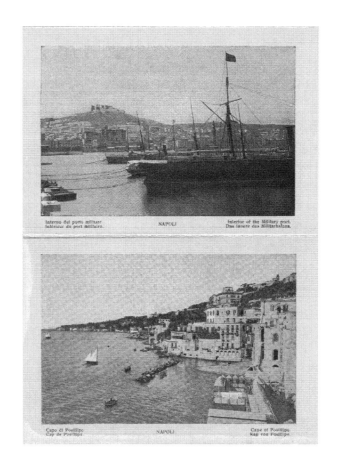

Interno del porto militare
Intérieur du port militaire.
NAPOLI
Interior of the Military port.
Das Innere des Militärhafens.

Capo di Posilipo
Cap de Posilipo
NAPOLI
Cape of Posilipo.
Kap von Posilipo.

Naples

We sailed in a 20,000 ton ship called the *Orama,* which in the end got sunk in the war, but it was the biggest ship going through the Suez Canal. All day I sat on deck. I could have gone to Cairo and caught it up at the other end but I stayed on the ship. I went through the canal sitting up there all day long.

Next I saw Port Said and there were loads of sharks swimming around the stern of the boat. As she went through, the waves were just lapping in the canal.

There was room for other little craft in the canal and in the middle there were these big lakes. There were no locks, you just went through the middle of these big lakes so the canal joined up the lakes I suppose. It took a day to go through so I missed Cairo but I couldn't have both. I didn't have much money anyhow, so if you couldn't spend any money there wasn't much point going ashore.

Then we came though to Naples.
'See Naples and die,' they say.
I don't know why they say that. We were there when Mussolini was alive – shhhh! Don't say anything about anything. Walls have ears. We got off at Naples but I never got to the disaster area about ten miles away where that volcano erupted at Mount Vesuvius where Pompeii got covered in lava, and where dogs and people were fossilised in this lava.

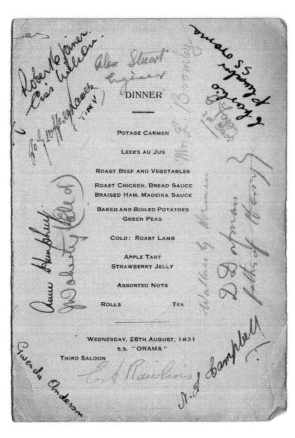

Signatures from the crew on the
last nigh

Norman's four friends

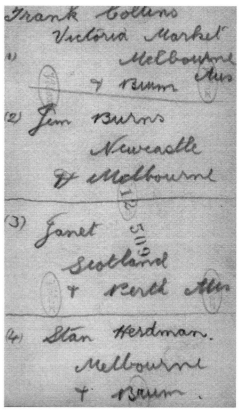

The Last Night

25th August 1931

They just put the mail off, nothing else at Plymouth and then we sailed up the English Channel. We had the last dinner and a dance and it was a nice, lively evening, our last evening on the boat.

The stewards and the table waiters used to do the entertainment. I've got a programme somewhere where they all signed their names for the last dinner. One of them had a saxophone. There was a pianist of course and a cornet player; only about three or four of them and they would just play all the dance tunes I like. It was done by the crew because they didn't have a special band.

That was ballroom dancing, waltzing, fox trot and quick step; that sort of thing. I used to like to watch it and I like Strictly Come Dancing now. They train them up but they don't play the old band music. I'm afraid that they don't play what I like anymore.

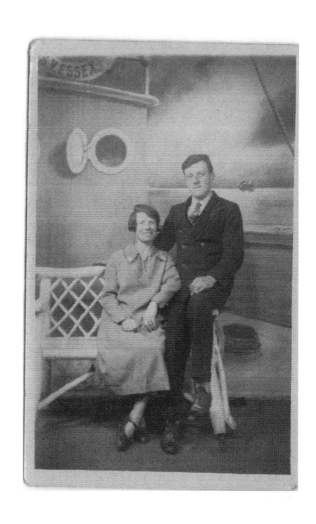

Norman and his mum pretending to be on the Orama
(In fact Norman says that it was a mock backdrop
but it looks realistic doesn't it?)

CHAPTER 17

Home at Last!

26th August 1931

I WAS SAD because it was all over I suppose, but I knew I was coming home and my mother was there to meet me at Tilbury, so I showed her all over the boat and everybody else drifted off.

I had a big bag with me and I got caught at customs where he undid the lot. I thought, good on you mate, you won't find anything in there but he insisted on going through it. Anyway, after that the crew said,

   'Yes, you can show yer mum over different parts of the ship,' so she saw where I'd been for six weeks.

Then we made our way home and I do remember coming up the road, because being in Australia everything was far and wide. When you came up here the road seemed so narrow. It was an avenue with trees overhanging the road and every branch of tree was almost touching in the middle. It was a nice avenue to drive up when I came home up the King's Road.

When we got home I think I just sat there on a chair in this back room until my dad came in from work and we met for the first time in four years and I suppose it was back to square one. There was no party. They were all out of work; no, it was a bad time then. I came home to help them with the bills but I couldn't get any work either.

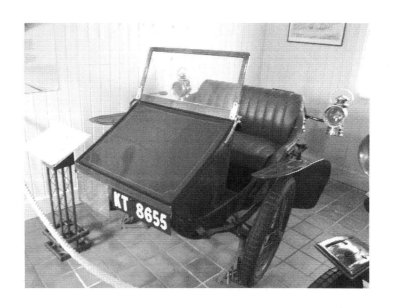

This unusual car is an AC Socialble
A three wheeler made when Norman's dad
worked there in 1911. It is on show at Brooklands.

My Dad had been working all the time I was away at AC Car Company, which stands for 'Auto Carriers7' at Thames Ditton. Sometimes he was on three days and then he was laid off for two or three weeks. Then they'd get busy again and have them back. They had them in and out as they wanted to; terrible time really. He was still making gear boxes for motor cars, but they were always going to go broke and in the end they did in 1930, just before I came back from Australia.

Then my dad was in and out of work all through the 30's. One week in this house we were all out of work and we had nothing coming in; only the dole which was fifteen and thruppence.

Mum said, 'What am I going to feed you on. I've got nothing.'
Then she had a brain wave.

She said, 'I know what I'll do,' and she made a suet pudding and cut it into four and we had that. That's what we ate for a week.

That was when I came home from Australia; when we had the 'out of work time.'

7. Auto Carriers Ltd, originally Autocars, moved to Ferry Works, Thames Ditton in 1911. After the war when it was, like many engineering works in the area, turned into a munitions factory, it became AC Cars in 1922 and went on to the most famous period in the company's history, gaining success in motor racing at Brooklands, Paris and Monte Carlo.

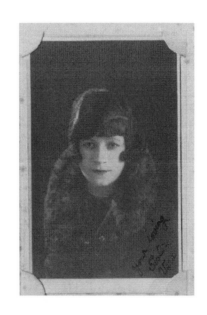

'Your Loving Sister Vera'

1932

I only had one sister, Vera, who died of pneumonia when she was only twenty one. That was a bit of a shock. I wasn't much use to any of them was I. In 1927 I went off to Australia and I came back in 1931 but she died at Christmas 1932.

During those two years I was out of work, except that I did the odd paper round and helped a bloke in his greengrocery business. I also did gardening jobs but nothing regular; anything I could get my hands on. I didn't get unemployment benefit though, because I'd been out of the country.
They said, 'You haven't paid anything in so you don't get anything out.'

You see, you had to work for six months before you were entitled to benefit. Then I worked for the rest of my life and never drew anything.

When I came home from Australia Mae was married. That was it. End of story. Of course, when I came back here Mae's sisters said to her,
'That Norman's back. Keep Mae away from him!'
I don't know whether they thought I was an ogre or something.
'Don't tell Mae,' they said.
What was that about? What did they think I'd do?
Then when Mae heard about my return they warned her,
'You mustn't get in contact with him.'

Then my dad was in work again but all the time he had a bad tummy and all he could eat was fish, but he never saw a doctor or anything. Once when I went up to Surbiton to get some fish for him, Mae was living in her mother and father-in-law's house in Fleece Road.
I saw her and I said, 'Oh hello Mae. How are you?'
'Oh she said. You can't talk to me 'cos I'm a married woman with a baby.'
So that was that so I said, 'Tara. San Fairy Ann.'
That was the only time I saw her at the time.

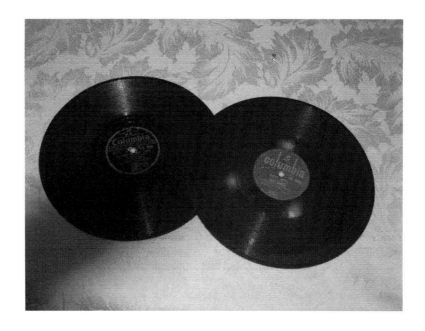

Columbia Records

8. Columbia Records, the oldest record label in the world, was founded in America in 1887 and The Columbian Gramophone Company was certainly the first to come to the UK in 1922, The label continued to produce records into the 1970's.

1932

We had electric installed in 1932. Before that we had gas lamps which came down from the ceiling and you had to light them. We had a gas lamp upstairs and in the front room too, but we never used them. We always used candles.

At that time they were now selling radios which you could run off your mains supply and they had to be earthed but my Dad said,

'You're not having one of them,' so we didn't have a new radio.

1933

I'd been home for two years and my mum got fed up.

She said 'I'm going to see one of your pals.'

'Don't do that,' Dad said.

'I'm going to see Mrs Thompson and I'm going to see if I can get you both into work.' and she did.

My dad was friendly with Mr Thompson, because they used to meet and have drinks together and so my mother got friendly with Mrs Thompson and her son-in-law was the foreman at Hawkers. You see my dad wouldn't go begging for work but Mum went anyway, so when she came back she said pointing to us,

'You and you have got jobs at Hawkers.' Ha ha. So I worked at Hawkers before I went to Australia and it was my first job when I came back.

Once I started work things improved but then the war came along, which was a tough time again of course. I never missed Australia. I'd done what I wanted to do really and I'd got over that. When you're young you want to do something different, prove something, prove to the street what you can do and I had to go away to Australia do it.

After a couple of years my dad got into a gramophone factory for a while; Columbias at Earlsfield, next door to Clapham Junction and he had to get there by train. He was there for a while working in maintenance called the millwright section and they looked after all the plant. You had the factory workers but you also had a maintenance department who maintained all the machinery. If anything went wrong then they put it right for the factory workers, who were making the actual records.

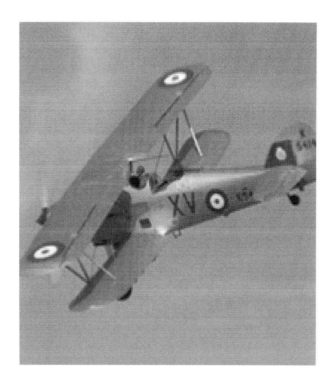

Hawker Hind 1935

CHAPTER 18

Hawkers

1933 - 1936

I WORKED IN Hawkers on the night shift where I was a Capstan machine operator making small things like nuts and bolts again; odds and ends for aircraft. Dad was in the tool room where they made jigs for parts of planes. There'd be a bracket and that'd be machined and it would fit in this jig and then they used to have holes to guide where to drill through it. That would be machined for parts of planes. You used to have to work to two tenths of a thou. That used to make me mad when they'd go and shoot it down. It was a wicked waste that was.

I was working there for six weeks and the foreman said,

'I've got to sack the night shift but I'll call for you in a week or two and get you on the day shift.'

That was the most terrible night, that last night. All the men were working and I couldn't say to them, 'In the morning you'll be sacked.'

The whole shift was sacked; that's how they used to treat them. I was standing in front of them. There was old Bill Long who lived down the road and I wanted to tell him.

'But you mustn't, mustn't, mustn't tell them,' the foreman had said. It had to be kept a secret, so all of them, the poor fellas, who went to work that night, they hadn't got a job in the morning. That was about forty workers; the whole night shift. Life wasn't too bad for me though. We were in work and we started to get a few things together. I was bringing in money; not a lot, about a pound or so.

Dad was bringing in about three pounds. Then they were building up for the war and when we started to work again in 1933, we were never out of work afterwards. All this time from then onwards it's got better and better. People might think they're badly off today but they've not been so well off in their lives; none of them. I don't care who they are. Mum and Dad started doing things, like they had the kitchen put in the scullery and the fireplace put in here and in the front room.

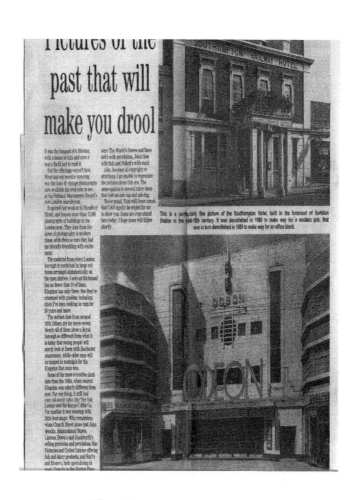

The Odeon Cinema Surbiton

In 1936 our next door neighbour came by.

He said, 'I've got a job as a steward over at Ravens Ait Island in the River Thames between Kingston and Surbiton. Do you want to buy my house?'

'How much do you want for it?' my Dad said.

'Three hundred pounds.'

So that's how we came to buy next door too, so we had two houses in 1936!

We had much more leisure time than we'd had before. The Sunday papers gave a review of what films were going to be released that week all over the country and down we went on a Monday evening, on the 601 Trolley Bus. These were busses on rails but they only lasted ten years; terrible waste that was. Anyway, we queued up outside waiting for the last show to come out.

In 1932 they had knocked down the old picture house and built this new Regal. It started off with Broadway Melody in about 1930, 1931 and it was in colour with actors like Gregory Peck and Joel Mc Kree. The talkies had arrived in Kingston on Thames. I remember watching Splinters of the Navy with Sydney Howard.

Then in the mid thirties Odeons were built everywhere and then in 1936 Granada came in. We used to go to the Empire on a Friday night and the Elite on a Thursday. My mother and sister would go to the first house and we'd be lined up for the evening show.

'What's it like,' we'd ask.

'Good,' they'd say as they passed us.

'Ok then,' we said, 'Ta, ta.'

That's how all the cinemas were born from 1931 to 1936 and they were all flourishing. We always dressed up to go out too. You never went in your ordinary clothes. You used to rush home from work, have something to eat, get all dressed up, shaved and off you'd go.

Of course after three years the war broke out.

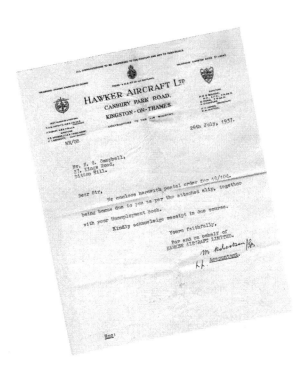

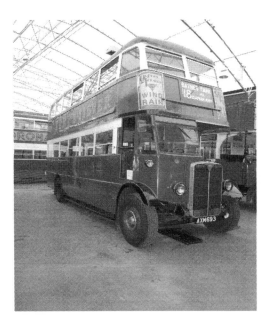

A local 1930's London Bus
118
In Brooklands Museum

CHAPTER 19

Meeting Peggy and Going to Bognor Regis!

1937

AT HAWKERS THERE was this girl always walking through the shop floor and all the boys used to wolf whistle and she used to just smile but she looked a nice girl. Then we had a works outing to Margate and I got together with this girl that day. She told me all about herself and that her mum often told her when she had to stay in and couldn't go out.

Anyway, she was sitting on my lap on the way back and we were kissing on the train. We'd had a few drinks you know! So that's how we got together. I took her out for a drink sometimes because I had a little car at the time.

This girl had a mate and so did I but he was already spoken for and I'd take him over Kew Bridge to see her on Sunday mornings, but he also picked up with my girl's mate and we sometimes went over to the Rose and Crown for a drink.

Once, my friend and these two girls were invited to go down to Margate in this big tent. I took my girl down in my car and another lodger took a lady called Peggy down in his car and we all went down in this big tent for a weekend and we had great fun.

On the way back my friend led the way but I missed him and took a wrong turning. Well, there was this guy from work in the other car and he was waving to my girl all the time. I thought, what's going on here. Then he pinched her off of me and that was that.

This man Bill, who was working with me at Hawkers, he introduced me to Peggy. We were going out to the pub drinking and I met her in this pub and we just got talking.

Peggy was running a boarding house and this bloke Bill, he was boarding there and she said to him,

'Bring your friend home to dinner.' So from Hawkers we used to go and have a dinner with Peggy. That's how it was and it went on from there.

Peggy looked after her mother but when she died she never wanted to work for anybody. She was very independent, so she started taking boarders. I think she worked on a meat stall in the market in Kingston on a Saturday night too.

Policy No. AS.2304582

SCHEDULE WITHIN REFERRED TO

| The Insured: | Name | NORMAN SPENCER CAMPBELL |
| | Address | 27 Kings Road Ditton Hill Surbiton |

| Date of signature of proposal and declaration | Period of Insurance | From the | Seventeenth day of August 1935 | Both dates inclusive |
| 17th August 1935 | | To the | Sixteenth day of August 1936 | |

| Annual Premium | £ 4 : 19 : 0 | Four Pounds Nineteen Shillings |) | Renewal date 17th August |

Index Mark and Registration Number	H.P. Treasury Rating	Make of Motor Car	Type of Body	Seating Capacity Including Driver	Year of Manufacture
MK 2015	9	SWIFT	Two Seater and Dickey	4	1926

Signed on the   Twentysecond   day of   August   One Thousand Nine Hundred and Thirty -five

Examined

CONDITIONS

Car Insurance for Norman's Swift 1936

122

So it started with me going back for dinner and that was it. We used to go out to the pubs mostly, because I had a friend who was a good pianist. He used to play at a pub over at Hampton Wick, the other side of the river to Kingston called the Crown and Anchor. He was a pianist in the cinema in the silent days and he had an opposite number, a woman who I got to know too, but he was a very good pianist. They used to say at Hawkers,

'Oh Vic, he can play all right.'

I thought, well these piano players, two a penny they are but we went on another Hawker's outing to Margate and coming back we called in at a pub where there was an old piano.

'Come on Vic,' they said

'Oh, I'm not playing,' he said.

In the end they got him to play. It was a really old piano, wanted tuning and the like, but when he got on that piano, he made it talk. Really talk.

Oh he can play, I thought. So I got quite friendly with him and he told me that he went over the Crown and Anchor on a Saturday and Sunday night to make ends meets. He had eight kids you see, and so he had a lot to keep going, so he earned himself five bob a night.

Then he used to play for a dance school for kiddies and at The Empire on a Saturday afternoon. He also had a little band of his own. He had a drummer, a cornet player and a violinist or something. There were about four of them. Very good they were.

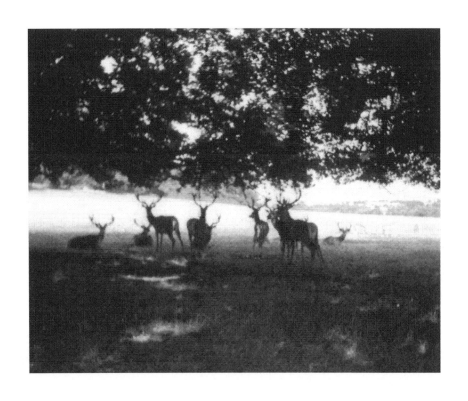

Richmond Park

One night he said,

'We've got a gig over at Fairey Aviation at Hayes, Middlesex. Do you think you could give us a lift?'

I had a little car then, a Swift, 'Yes sure,' I said.

So I picked Vic up. There was the base player who sat on the dicky seat and I got the other two in the side of me and I remember that it was perishing cold; frost on the ground in an open top car. I remember that. So we had a dance and a laugh that night. Vic went wherever he could get a few bob to keep things going. It was a hard time for him but that was what it was like through the thirties.

Of course I was still going down to lunch at Pegg's and looking back I think that's what happened. Pegg caught me on the rebound. It just gelled again somehow. We weren't together long before we got married, Peggy and me. I was in her house one day and she asked me to marry her. She just said she wanted me. Of course she was older than I was as well. I was twenty seven and she was thirty seven.

That night I said to my Mum,

'I'm getting married to this woman Peggy and she's older than me.'

'Fetch her over here,' Mum said.

After my Dad had met Peggy he said, 'I don't want you to marry her. She's far too old.'

So then I had to tell Pegg, 'We can't get married. My Dad doesn't want us to.'

Pegg said, 'Well, I'll commit suicide then.'

So Pegg and I went up to Richmond Park and sat on a seat for quite some time and she said again, 'If we don't get married then I'll commit suicide.'

She'd fallen for me you see; much more her way than me.

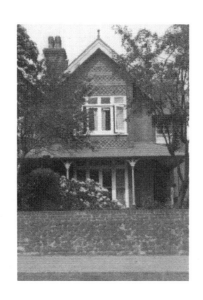

Norman and Peggy's House in Bognor Regis

So next I had to come back home and tell my Mum and Dad.

'She wouldn't do that,' my Dad said.

'I'm sure she would,' I said. I could tell. It was more she grabbed me than I grabbed her. I don't know why. She fell for me and that was it.

I upset all the family at the time. My cousin was very close and she wouldn't have it.

'She's too old for you,' she said and she cut me off altogether. That was the cousin who had given me the ring that I lost on the journey to Australia. Anyway she came round years later.

So in '37 I left home when I got married. In the end only my Mum and Dad came to the wedding which we had in Chichester. Now there's another story. My other Grandma, she lived at Bognor.

'We'll get married and go and live down in Bognor and get a boarding house,' Pegg said.

So I was getting led all the time. I wasn't doing anything. I mean I shouldn't chuck in a good job up and go to Bognor should I, but I went along with it anyway.

Also my Grandma said, 'I want you down here. It'll be company for me.'

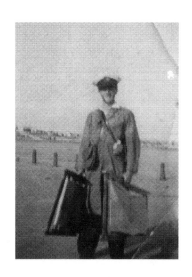

Norman ~ the cheerful
deck-chair attendant!

So that was it. We got married on 10th July 1937 in the registry office in Chichester. I drove me and Pegg and my Mum and Dad down there and they were the only witnesses. That was all. We got married on the 10th and Pegg's birthday was on the 11th.

I remember my Dad bought half a dozen oranges. I don't know why. Half a dozen oranges. Ha, ha!

Pegg just wore an ordinary Sunday dress. It was just the law to go through the ceremony to register the marriage, so that was how it was done. In the end we got on quite well. and we had forty one years together. That's not a bad is it?

In Bognor we had an ordinary house but Pegg knew what to do to set up a boarding house, but we were a good distance away from the sea. Anyway, we put a notice up and we got people coming in and people came down from here too and stayed for a holiday. So it went along like that.

I couldn't get work at first so I got a job on the council on the deck chairs. It was a lovely summer for me. It was like a holiday.

Of course when the summer was over there was no more of that and so Pegg said,

'I'm going down to the police station to see if I can get any coppers.'
So she got three coppers boarding. That went along until November and these coppers kept on changing because they had to go off to different places.

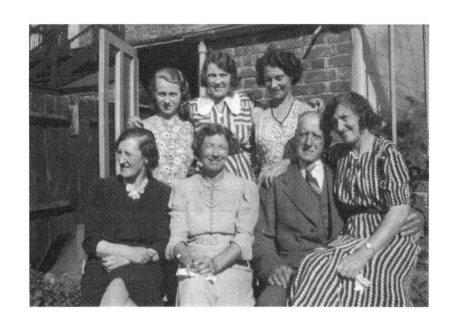

Peggy top second left and some of her lodgers

1938

I still couldn't get a job and so I said,

'It's hopeless me getting a job down here.'

And so she said, 'Right, pack up then. We'll go back to Kingston,' just like that.

So we went back to Kingston in '38 and of course there was plenty of work in my line, so we got a place at Lower Ham Road in Kingston; thirty bob a week it was.

I went to see one of my mates.

'Yer,' he said. 'We'll get you a job up at Parnells in Chessington.'

It was a new factory started up in Oakcroft Road, getting ready for the war.

There was a factory that had come up from Bristol; extended from the Bristol factory. There was another one that built tanks next door and another one that made diving equipment. They were all on war work. Of course they were coming round with gas masks when we came back, so we were all issued with a gas mask which was in 1938.

We set up a boarding house straight away and we got people from Hawkers and Bentalls; plenty of people. I was up at Parnells for a while and they didn't have any rigid night and day work. If you were on day work, you were on day work, but if a bloke on the night shift wanted a change you could do it. They'd allow you to.

So I had been up there for about six months or so and this bloke on nights said,

'Could you give us a break for about four or five weeks.'

'Yer, ok, I'll give you a break,' I said, but the devil wouldn't come back and so I was left on night work.

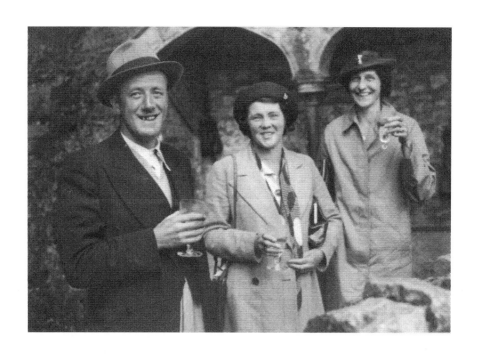

Peggy and friends on holiday

June 1939

The workers were always after more money and so those blokes I'd been working with at Hawkers said,

'There's a little factory over near Malden we'll try.'

Of course, all these little factories wanted to get workers. LC Engineering was doing subcontract work, so I went over there and they said,

'Yes, we'll start you off at one and six an hour.'

Well, that was thru pence a week more than Parnells, so I was a setter operator there, making nuts and bolts for planes again. That was in 1939 and I was there throughout the war.

I went to LC Engineering in June 1939 but I said to the bloke,

'I've booked a holiday for a fortnight and I'm taking me holiday.'

'Oh that's sensible. That'll be all right,' he said.

We set off on our way to Dawlish camping but a spring in my car broke going down some high ridges. We were on this hill and there was a bloke who helped me to steer on to the verge. He released the brake but the poor man got all smothered in oil and grease helping us.

It was our first holiday but instead of going to Dawlish, we turned round and went back to Weymouth. That was the first fortnight's holiday we ever had.

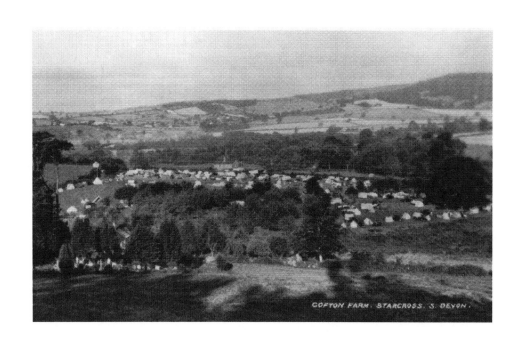

Happy Holidays in Devon!

After that we always went camping in Dawlish. We started with a tent and we drifted up to caravans and then to hotels. We climbed the ladder over the years. We went down there seventeen years running. You see, there was this farm which took dogs and you couldn't get dogs in everywhere.

Other guests came from the Midlands and we got to know them and I'm still corresponding with some people at Christmas from those days. Unbelievable! So we used to make some good friends in the old camping days. A lot of them have died of course. That's years ago you see. You get too old and you lose them.

At home we were always shifting house and Pegg said one day,

'I went round to see a house down Richmond Road today and we're gonna move down there.'

'What for?' I asked.

She gave a reason but I don't remember what it was, so we moved down there for about six months. We were only renting because I never bought anything. It's always come to me. Anyway, we paid two bob extra for a garage which was good.

Now we're settled, I thought. We're in 33 Staunton Road and we're settled. And we were; we were there for nineteen years, all through the war. We moved there in 1939, the same time as I got that job. I had one of those occupations when you were conscripted but in a different way.

We had people as boarders from all over the country. Peggy was a grafter, always paper hanging and painting, always on the go. She was strange really but we had our good times. Peggy couldn't have any children but I never wanted any either.

Surrey Comet 1939

CHAPTER 19

The War Years

1939 – 1945

MY MOTHER USED to say,

'All these people having children. They're just breeding gun fodder.'
You see, in our time it was always about wars and talk about wars. That's all I heard while I grew up. That was real. I mean, there were millions killed. Terrible it was. You saw a lot of the youngsters and all they wanted to do was to fight. They wanted to go to war. Today they're breaking out in riots because they've got nothing better to do because they want to be in the action.

There was that fatal morning when Mr ... was it Macmillan. No, it was a doddering old Birmingham family who were very rich. They ran politics. Mr Chamberlain, that's who it was. Well, just before that he came home waving a bit of paper yelling,

'Peace in our time.'

He'd been over to have a word with Adolf. It wasn't very long after that Hitler kept on invading all over the continent and then he went into Poland. We were supposed to protect Poland so that was it. If we didn't get an answer that Hitler'd refrain from entering Poland then we'd be at war at midday that day.

We heard it on the radio on 3rd September. That's that. We were at war. For the first year it was just a phoney war. Nothing much went on. Hitler was getting on with it over there, consolidating all Europe, then of course when he invaded France we really had to act.

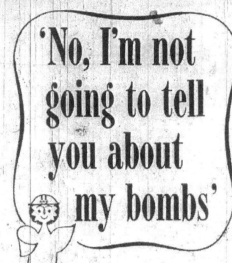

'No, I'm not going to tell you about my bombs'

Speaking for the 15 Gas Companies set out below, I want to thank Londoners for their patience and understanding.

For reasons of National Security we cannot tell you all the difficulties involved in keeping London's gas supply going.

But we can tell you something of what we are doing to deal with the problems caused by air raids.

These Companies have pooled their resources of men and equipment and have established the London Regional Gas Centre.

Day and night, gas is being made at more than 50 Gas Works, and thousands of men are standing by ready to go out to tend the 14,000 miles of mains and the 3 million meters that supply gas to homes and factories.

These men have their own casualty list from enemy action — their own record of gallantry — their own recipients of the George Medal.

Whatever the New Year may bring, these Companies will spare no effort individually and collectively to see that your gas supply is maintained.

THE LONDON REGIONAL GAS CENTRE HAS BEEN ESTABLISHED BY

Barnet District Gas & Water Company	North Middlesex Gas Company
Commercial Gas Company	South Metropolitan Gas Company
Croydon Gas Company	South Suburban Gas Company
East Surrey Gas Company	Tottenham & District Gas Company
The Gas Light & Coke Company	Uxbridge, Maidenhead, Wycombe & District Gas Company
Hampton Court Gas Company	
Hornsey Gas Company	Wandsworth & District Gas Company
Lea Bridge Gas Company	Watford & St. Albans Gas Company

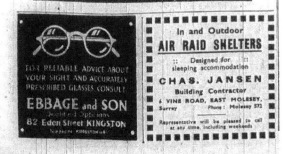

We were on war work back home.

Pegg said, 'You're gonna be conscripted so I'm not gonna work for anybody else. I'm doing war work looking after these people who've been drafted in. I'm doing my bit.'

Then she said, 'Not only that but, if we don't have these people they're going to draft soldiers on to me in the night.'

She was right because we were right behind the barracks.

So I said, 'You're doing the right thing girl.'

The war years were terrible really; you just worked, ate and slept. All your life was really in your factory. It was a twelve hour shift 8 'til 8; day shift and night shift; twelve hours on and twelve hours off. You'd go home to eat and and try and sleep but then there was a run of those air raids.

At first they had shelters in 1939 in the playing fields. Then they came round with an Anderson shelter you could dig in your garden, but we didn't get one of those. At first we just went under the stairs if the sirens went off, when you got an air raid warnings in the road.

Everyone was forced to be a volunteer to take a watch at night. They took me to this place but I told them, 'Get lost' They put you on a watch at 2 to 4 in the morning.

Pegg said, 'You're not getting any rest. You can't do that.'

So other people did the fire watch and I got out of that.

FOOD FACTS

GOOD RESOLUTIONS

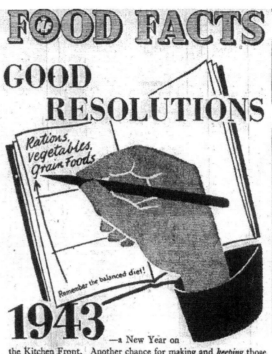

Rations, vegetables, grain foods

Remember the balanced diet!

1943—a New Year on the Kitchen Front. Another chance for making and *keeping* those good resolutions of yours.

You've always planned to take up all your allowance of Household Milk and Dried Egg. You've always meant to make use of your full cheese ration. You've always intended to eat potatoes instead of bread. You've often thought of serving more vegetables.

Well, here again is your opportunity to do all those things you've always meant to do on the food front. You make the resolutions, follow the method given here, and you'll keep them in 1943.

POET'S CORNER

Auntie threw her rinds away.
  To the lock-up she was taken.
There she is and there she'll stay
  Till she learns to save her bacon.

•

When in winter Nature limits what the *cows* hold
Your trusty grocer helps you out with ' Household '.

•

Don't waste fuel
On a vegetabuel;
It's more to your credit
To shred it.

**LISTEN TO
THE KITCHEN FRONT
EVERY MORNING
AT 8.15**

1943 IN THE KITCHEN :—

1 See that each one of the family has his own full rations, and remember this includes Dried Egg and Household Milk. Make the most of your cheese ration.

2 Eat at least 1 lb. of potatoes every day. Don't peel them. Cook them in their skins. They are better for you and tastier, too.

3 Eat plenty of green vegetables and salads, and when you can't get greens eat root vegetables, especially swedes and carrots.

4 Cook your vegetables the modern way. Use very little boiling water. Shred or slice your vegetables first. Cook very quickly with the lid on. Eat as soon as cooked.

1943 IN THE SHOPS :—

5 Do your shopping in as few bits as possible. It will save the shopkeeper's time and paper. Try and buy a week's supply of goods at one time. This isn't easy for you, but your shopkeeper, who is very short-handed, will be very grateful.

6 Take paper or piece of cloth to wrap your shopping in. Especially save paper at the butcher's whenever possible.

7 Always return milk bottles well rinsed and don't forget to save the milk bottle caps for the milkman.

1943 IN THE LARDER :—

8 Don't throw away a scrap of food. Bits of left-over fish or vegetables make splendid sandwich fillings. Odds and ends of bread can be used in puddings. Use cheese rind for flavouring sauces. Shred the outside leaves of cabbages and use them in soups and stews.

9 Don't hoard your Dried Egg. It is meant to be used now. Keep it in a dry cool place.

10 Don't forget to ask for your Household Milk at the grocer. And read the instructions on the tin before you use it.

THE MINISTRY OF FOOD, LONDON, W.I.   FOOD FACTS No. 130

Then I got into the Dad's army; I got drafted into that instead, but I got into trouble about drill.

I said, 'How can I get to drill if I've not come home from work? You're just packing up when I finish.'

So I got out of that too but at weekends I used to go on guard up at the lock at Teddington. I used to spend Saturday nights up there on guard. Then there was a Sunday once a month at six o'clock in the morning, you had to go down Shepperton way, down the river, to have a drill for The Home Guard, then back to work at eight on Monday morning.

They used to say, 'Did you hear that bombing last night?'

'I didn't hear a thing,' I said. 'I went out like a light.'

I used to go bang out. I just couldn't keep my eyes open.

1944

Well, towards the end of the war, Mr Morrison invented another air raid shelter. It was a metal table really, which had steel girders for legs with wire mesh on the sides. It was sat up in the corner of the room and if anything came down, this metal thing should stand the weight.

The dogs used to go under it, so when the old sirens went, we used to get under that towards the end of the war when the doodlebugs used to come over. That was in 1944.

You see, when the war was nearly over, Hitler started bringing out a lot of new things. There was that doodlebug and the V2 that went up and it didn't do surface damage like the buzz bomb. Those were pilotless aircraft which pushed tiles up and blew out glass over a large area.

But when the V2 came down, where there were houses only a large crater would be left. It was pulverised to nothing; people, furniture, nothing, just a hole. They were terrible. Of course if you heard them then you were all right; but if you didn't hear one. We live through some terrible times. It was another push to see if they could ruin us.

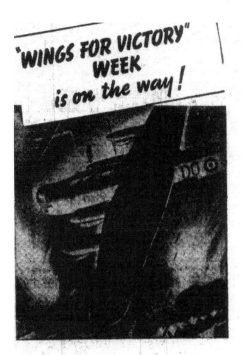

'WINGS FOR VICTORY' WEEK is on the way!

You remember last year's Warship Week —and the War Weapons Week of the year before? This year, in tribute to the Royal Air Force, an even greater nation-wide War Savings Drive will sweep the Kingdom —"Wings for Victory" Week.

London leads the way—its Week opens on March 6th. Its aim is to save and invest £150,000,000. This calls for the greatest War Savings effort that we've ever made. The target for your district is set by your Local Savings Committee and will count towards London's total. Your Committee is already at work. Give it your support! Help your district to get its target. In this way it will secure its own "Victory Wings." At the same time it will make a valuable contribution to the whole London effort.

The London Wings for Victory Week covers the following areas: London and all Metropolitan Boroughs, County of Middlesex and the Essex Boroughs of Barking, East Ham, West Ham, Leyton, Ilford & Walthamstow

WIN YOUR VICTORY WINGS
MARCH 6-13

Issued by the National Savings Committee

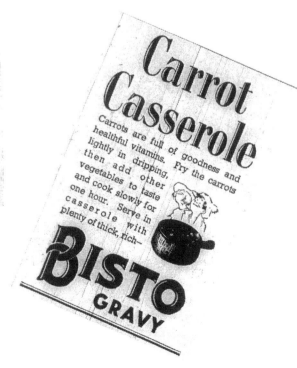

We did better than most by having more people in the house. Pegg could fiddle around a bit and also she was a good one to get in with the shop keepers and so she used to get extra rations. She was good like that; very good with food. The only thing was that you could never get any eggs. We had this reconstituted egg from America instead. Horrible!

We had this one old bloke lodging and he said, 'I'm not eating that.'

Pegg said, 'If you don't eat that you can go without.'

So he said, 'That's all I got at the last place.'

'That's all you'll get at any place,' I said. 'That's all we've got.'

So other than that, the worst thing was that you lived at work so you were with your work mates more than anybody else and you got very friendly with them. I was a setter, a tool setter with five women. I set up the machines and they did the work.

There was one girl I was quite friendly with, you know; you're pushed into these things working with them all the time and we got quite intimate. Then I came in one morning and I saw a group just standing over there, so I looked over and I thought, hello, what's going on.

Then someone said, 'you'll have to go over and tell him.'

So a woman came over and she said, 'She got killed last night.'

Do you know, I don't know what it was, but something went dead in me when they told me she was dead and I never laughed again for three months. That upset me quite a bit. Maybe I was in love with her. Who knows, but it was just that we were thrown together. The other four I wasn't bothered about but I remember this particular one. I remember how hard it was when she... well, there you are. That's the way it goes. Kathy her name was. We were pretty close. That was February '44 when Kathy got killed.

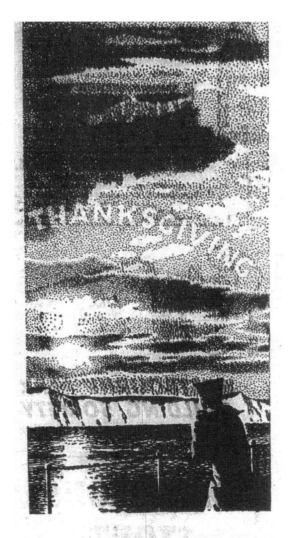

INTO HARBOUR! A great day has dawned.

With our hearts filled with thankfulness for

victory, let us make this great resolve!—

Let us continue by our thrift and savings

to make a land free from anxiety and want.

Let us prove that the sacrifices of war have

not been in vain.

GIVE THANKS BY SAVING

Tragedy and Finality

Then there was young boy. He was in an air raid shelter made of cement but one of the girders broke in half and it fell on his chest and killed him. Poor little devil.

Then there was another boy. He was dead keen to get into the Air Force and he got called up. He served his time, got his training but on his first bombing trip out to Germany he got killed. His first trip!

May 1945

We knew a year before that it was coming to an end, but on May 8th we heard it on the wireless. I remember me and old Murray were sitting on the curb outside the house talking and then later on there was a chap who used to work at Hawkers and they had a bonfire down the bottom of our road. After that Jock and I went up to London and saw the parade. An amazing feeling although we were a bit numb too.

It all changed then. At the factory we were packing up because they were short of work for us and then they gave us the sack because they didn't want to build any more planes.

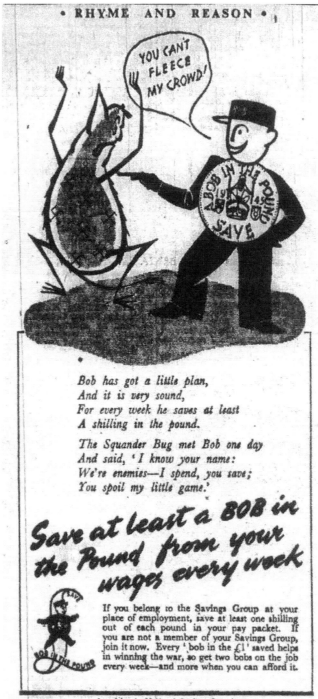

1945/46

This would be before I went to Decca so it must have been soon after '45.
Pegg knew I'd been to Australia and I suppose I talked about it a lot, I don't
know. Anyway a lot of people went there after the war and so we applied for a
berth to Australia and at first they came back to us and said that all the shipping
had been destroyed during the war but they said,

'We'll put you on a list and when your turn comes around we'll get in
touch with you.'

So I said to Pegg, 'We'll have to leave it at that.'

Well, it must have been a couple of years later, when I'd started to work at
Decca that they said, 'We now have a berth if you are still interested.'

I'd got settled in down at Decca by then and Peggy had gone off the idea
and so we just stayed here. If we'd have gone straight away we would have
done it, but as it was we'd got settled in here. Mind you Peggy would have done
anything for a bit of excitement or a challenge. She was that way inclined. She
always wanted to do something new. She wanted to have our own business and
that was another story.

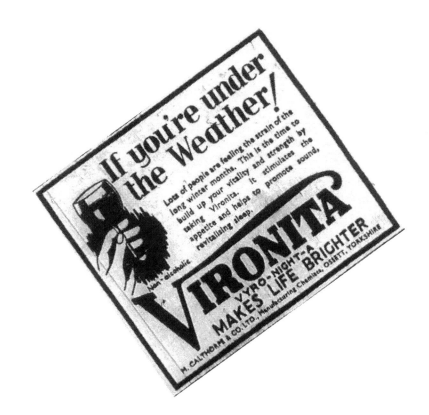

One day she said,

'There's a shop advertised in Norwood. Can we go over and see it?'
I wasn't all that keen and so I said,

'Yes all right,' just to pacify her and I drove us there but the shop was
almost empty. They kidded us into buying it. It wasn't a lot of money but there
was nothing there so I started to think; you'd got to stock it all up.

'That's useless,' I said when I got back home. 'How are we gonna do
anything with a place like that. You can see they just want to get out of it.

'There's not much in it Pegg. This deal is off. I'm ringing them up and
I'm gonna say no.'

Pegg still said, 'Well, we could try.'

But I said, 'No, that's off,' and that's what I did.

I don't know what sort of mess we would have got into there, but I couldn't
see any future in it. So I did put my foot down sometimes.

I mean I tried. I went to Australia and tried everything on my own. It was an
adventure and I was all for that but this time I had reservations and so I
stopped it. She saw no further than what she saw then. She didn't look to the
future.

It all worked out right in the end though. It was all up and down at times
but mostly it was enjoyable.

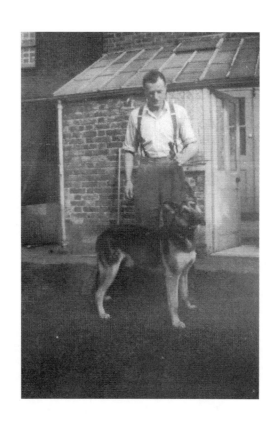

Norman and Queenie

CHAPTER 20

It's a Dog's Life!

1944 - 1948

WE HAD OUR first an Alsatian in 1944 called Flash, but we had to have her put down so we got a puppy from New Malden in 1947 called Queenie. In fact she was registered as Queen of Rodmark. All these dogs were pedigree and they were registered at the kennel club. Then we met a fellow and his wife when we were exercising up by the common and we knew they had an Alsatian too.

'We're making a few bob out of breeding from her,' he said. 'We get seven to ten pound a pup.'

So we thought, that's a good idea; we'll get a few bob that way too.

I used to go to the dog shows and I took particular notice of one dog who was a lovely looking animal who was always taking prizes, so we decided to get Queenie mated with this dog and we got in touch with the fellow.

'Yes,' he said, 'bring her over.'

We took her there and he said,

'We'll just leave them together and we'll go and have a cup of tea.'

We stayed there for a while but Queenie wouldn't have anything to do with it! We took her back home but when her time came she had a false pregnancy and she would imagine she was having pups. We didn't know what to do so we went back to the man and he said,

'I'll tell you what. There's a nice puppy we've got for sale.'

So we bought another puppy and that's how we got Penny for seven pound. So that's how we came to have two Alsatians. That was in about 1948.

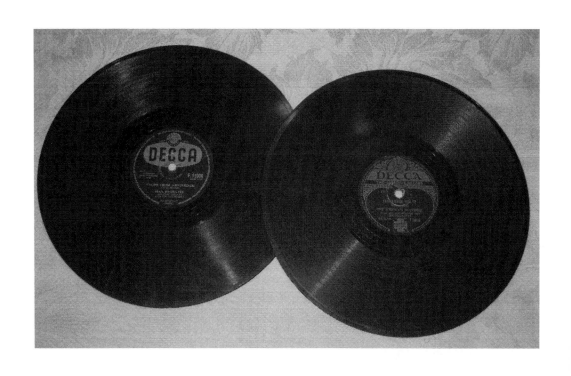

Decca gramophone records

CHAPTER 21

Decca 'It's all Right Now!'

March 1st 1948.

AT THE END of the war, nobody wanted any war planes. In fact the industry was dying down from '44 onwards. We were trying to get any sort of work that was going around. I went back to being a Setter Operator and I stayed there for a while.

Then the foreman said, 'I don't know. I just can't get enough work so I'll have to let you go.'

So I packed up; I'd had enough anyway. At that time you had to report to the Labour Exchange because you were still under their direction even though the war was over. When you changed jobs you had to go through them.

'Try Leylands,' the chap said.

'What's the point of trying there,' I said. 'They're all the same. They don't want anybody.'

'Try 'em,' he said but I went up there and they didn't want anybody. I went back and was sent to a couple of places but they were the same.

'I'll tell you what,' he said. 'If you can find your own job, then we'll release you.'

So I looked around and I had always wanted to get into Decca. My Dad was in Columbia for some while before the war and he said that it was good to get into the record business.

At that time he worked at Projectiles. He'd never wanted to work there, because it was right close to where he lived, but in the end he finished his time up at Projectiles.

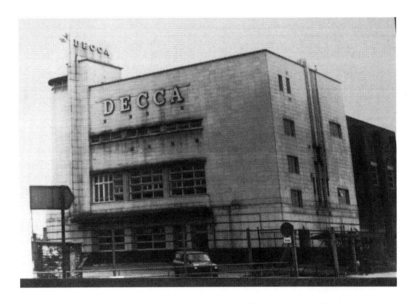

The Decca factory in Burlington Road, New Malden

10. Decca was one of the greatest employers in the area with a workforce of 700, making up to 60,000 records a day but making radar during World War Two. Artists signed to Decca in the 1930s and 1940s included Louis Armstrong, Billie Holiday, The Andrews Sisters, Judy Garland, Billy Cotton and Guy Lombard amongst others.

So I got this job at Decca₁₀ in New Malden. It was a new career for me and I earned 2 shillings per hour plus two pence cost of living bonus; that's what they called it.

At Decca I worked in the plating and finishing shop. We were making dies really; they called them a family. The bands recorded music up at the studio in North London somewhere, then it would come down on a disc to us. First we'd get a copy off of that disc. It was only a wax copy, or at least it was at first.

From the disc from the studio we grew what we called the Master, a silver faced master, which took about 24 hours to grow in copper baths and so you got your Master. Next you grew your Positive. As a family they called the Positive the Mother. On the Master the lines were up but when you grew the Positive the lines were down, like grooves. From your Mother you started producing children which went to the press.

Also, they didn't want to use the Master again if possible, so that was all greased up and put away, but occasionally they had to go back to the original. We also grew a Copy Master to put in store, so that if you wanted any more Positives you grew them from the Copy. We were exporting Positives to other countries all over the world so that they could produce the records themselves.

When you had produced your family you had to produce one side and then the other side so that you had two stampers in the press to get one record. They stamped the records in a different department. Our job was to produce the tools to produce the record.

At that time it was all shellac records; a ten inch and a twelve inch record; two sides an A side and a B side. It was all done in copper. The trouble was you couldn't grow a flat plate. It would be twice as thick on the outside as it was in the middle.

In the machine shop they made the dies that hold the stampers which had to be flat. They used to swing it in the bath, hanging vertically downwards, but then we got a rotary which turned around and it was quicker to grow it that way, when we used to turn the back of them so they were flat. There was one vat of copper solution and the plate you were growing was screwed on to a spindle, which was put down and you rotated it horizontally. This was so that the chap who made the dies would get two flat plates.

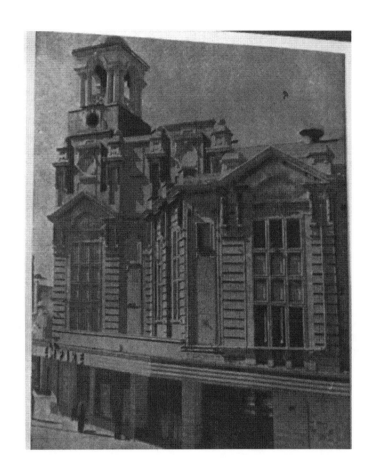

Kingston Empire 1948

1949

After twelve months in '49 I got dermatitis, which was the danger with plating. You see, it was over 40 degrees which is 100 odd Fahrenheit, with steam coming off of the vats and it affected my skin so I started scratching.

The foreman said, 'There's nothing we can do about it. If you stop in here you'll only get worse. You'd better find yourself a job on a farm, out in the fresh air.' He paused and said, 'I know what I can do, I'll make you up into a charge hand.'

Fortunately the opposite number to me on nights didn't want to go on days and so I was on permanent days. When I was a charge hand I did a lot of overtime because I had to meet the man from the night shift.

My manager said, 'Tell him what you do.'

So I met Bert at the beginning of his shift, because they used to do different things at night. I used to stay on 'til about eight o'clock or half past eight sometimes just jawing. By that time I'd reached twenty pounds a week and I'd reached £1,000 a year mark!

I saw lots of changes at Decca. At first they had a long bath and they grew the plates in copper with a rotary hanging vertically along the bath. The copper ones took four and a half hours to grow.

Next they decided to grow the plates in nickel instead of growing them in copper, so that was another job we had to learn. They were all in the bath and hanging vertically in a rocking movement growing six on each side, so you had a dozen in the vat.

Another invention they made, which was quicker of course, was four banks with nickel solution. It was all done electrically under amp hours and they took 200 amps, so we grew one plate in an hour. We had four banks of six, that's twenty four plates! So they did away with everything else. There were improvements all the time I was there, so it was always interesting.

As we went on, it kept on improving. First we produced Mono and then Stereo.

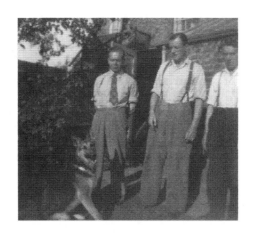

Queenie, our Alsatian enjoyed the company of our lodgers

CHAPTER 22

The Tale of Many Lodgers

Early 50's

PEGGY TOOK LODGERS up at Kingston and your dad was one of the last lodgers. I would never have met you through your father, but it was your mother. She wanted to see where your father lived and Peggy and Pat took to each other. They got on very well and from then on they kept in contact. I didn't go to your mum and dad's wedding but I went to Christine's, your sister's.

We visited your mum and dad when they first got married though. They had two flats, the first at Sanderstead and the second in Croydon. We first went up there in 1953 and there was a little bridge and a little stream. That's how we started visiting you at Christmas time, when your mum and dad were first married. Your mum used to draw me a map. We got to the North Road and there were two branches.

'Up that way,' she said.

Then they went in for the house at Warlingham and we went over there quite often. One Sunday we were just sat in the road and there were people coming out, going to your sister's Christening; your Grandmother and Grandfather Green and your other Grandmother and Grandfather Jackson and your Nan, I met her too, your Mum's Grandmother! Of course your grandfather died young.

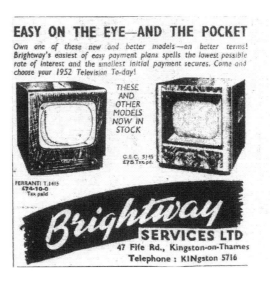
Surrey Comet 1953

160

I'd been in Decca about eight years and I was working all the hours God sends, so I didn't see much, but in '53 we'd just broken into television. The Kingston Empire cinema started advertising them. called myself one of the pioneers and I got this set in Staunton which we had it in time for that wedding; Princess Elizabeth's. All the street wanted to come to see the wedding. It was only a small thing, a nine inch, but it had a magnifier on it.

The television cost £50 or you could rent it for so much a month and then at the end of the term you could buy it. I thought about it and since I was spending so much in the Kinema and so much in the Elite and so much in the Empire, I thought that all of it could go to pay for the television instead and then we didn't have to go out.

We'd have all our entertainment indoors; magic. But that was the worst thing that could ever happen. All our social life went. I've never been out to the pictures since. The other thing is that everyone is scruffy these days. No one ever dresses up anymore. And then many of the picture houses were turned into Bingo halls when television took over.

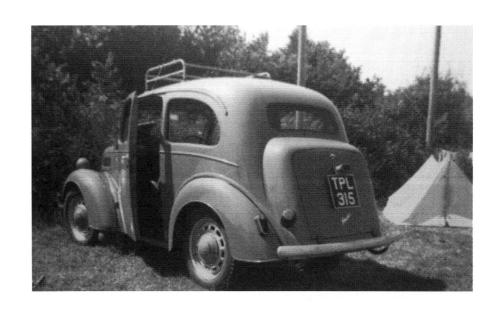

Norman's Ford Popular 1953

1953

After the war in '53 I also started off with a new car. I decided I didn't want anymore second hand cars but there were no cars being produced 'cos all the car industry had been turned over to the war effort.

There was a chap at work who told me to apply for a car. You would have to wait in order and it would be about twelve months before you got one. He paid someone in the queue one hundred pounds extra so that he got a car straight away. I thought I wouldn't do that, but that year I went to the Motor Show.

They'd produced this Popular, they called it. Just some nuts and bolts; there wasn't much in it. The inside was lined with stuff like hardboard, that's all; no carpets on the floor and all the draft came through the boards. There was no heater and you always had your windows down to make hand signals. There was only one red light on the back; that was all.

I had this Popular and it was a good buy. I think it was only about four hundred quid. He said it'd hold its price. Everybody was envious of it, and I suppose and I had it for seven years and it was still worth a lot so I thought I'd trade it in.

This man said,
        'I'll give you one hundred pounds more than you get for it.'
I was going to trade it in and they offered me one hundred and fifty for it. I thought that's not a bad price after I'd had it for seven years, so I said to this chap,
        'You can have it for one hundred and eighty,' so I sold it to him.

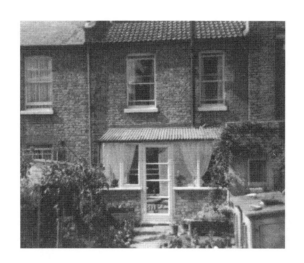

Home again

CHAPTER 23

Back to the Family Home

1955

IN 1955 MY Mother died and my poor old Dad, he was getting... well he was only 76 but he was worn out, the poor devil. They used to work long hard hours and then of course there were all the 'out of work' times too. I don't know. We used to come up to see him and he would clean the fire out but it'd take him all day to do it.

One day he said, 'I wish you'd come up here and stay with me.'
So we had to make up our minds.
Pegg said, 'I can make your Dad's house into a little palace.'
'Hang on a minute,' I said. 'Are you sure you're going to do this; look after my Dad, help him up and things. If you're sure, you have to make a commitment that you will look after him.'
She said, 'I'll do it.'
I was worried because Pegg often said she wanted to do this and then she wanted to do that and then she wanted to be off again. So I said that if we're going to move in with Dad, then that's it. Otherwise I wouldn't have come back. I would have had to put Dad into a home or something.

1956

We had the bathroom put in in '56 before we came up here and we installed a boiler instead of the old copper, for hot water. At first we brought down a fire that used to be on all day with a hob, but it smoked a lot and so we had a gas fire put in the back room here and in the living room too.

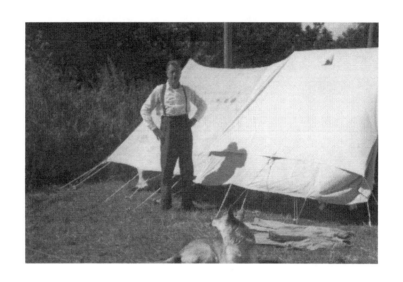

Here we are camping in Star Cross, Dawlish
This is Penny one of our Alsatians

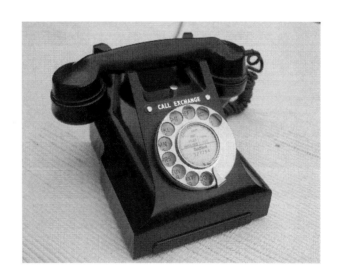

That's the first time I ever got Pegg settled really, but we didn't take in any lodgers here. Pegg did all the decorating and gardening and, true to her word, she looked after Dad. All my life was spent at Decca and there wasn't much life at home for us, but we used to have weekends and we got away for two weeks each year, still at Starcross in Dawlish.

Mrs Trenchard, who lived two doors away, had been neighbours for years and so she looked after Dad, getting him some bread, or whatever he wanted and I rang him up every other night. I had to come through about three exchanges to get here; murder it was. Now, today, you just press a button and you're through to Australia.

We used to have a picnic sometimes on a Sunday at Worthing or Brighton. We always used to get out at weekends, though not so much in the winter time. That's when we used to visit your Mum and Dad.

Penny

I think we brought Penny up to your Mum and Dad's as well, I'm sure we did. We had her for thirteen years. I don't know how your Dad came to lodge with us with two Alsatians. That I'll never know. This is Penny on one of our camping trips.

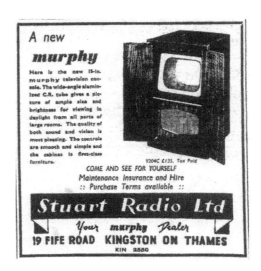
Surrey Comet 1958

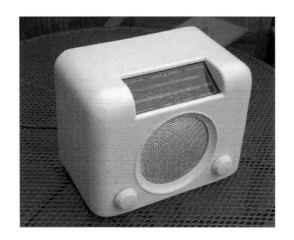

CHAPTER 24

TV Pioneer

1958

WHEN WE MOVED in with Dad I progressed along to another television but that wasn't very successful, although I wasn't here much at night. I only had a couple of hours in the evenings. There was only one station actually, the BBC.

Then this bloke came up and he said, 'This is a better set.'

And we said, 'Here we go again.'

We bought it though, but that didn't last long either and then I got another one which was a Consul; it was quite a nice screen. They kept saying that they were building a new mast but then we got a Post Office link.

There were some good programmes on, I remember. We had stories and excerpts from the London theatres and some really good drama series, but more often than not the programme broke down. Then all you got on the screen was a potter's wheel or fishes in a tank for a couple of hours. This set was alright but then it started to fade and fade away, so I said to the electrician that it must be losing its signal.

'No way,' he said, 'It can't lose a signal.'

'But it does,' I said.

'Ok,' he said. 'I've got a friend who knows something about televisions. I'll get him to come and have a look at it.'

This chap said, 'Instead of 240 you can knock it down to 230 and you'll get your picture through better.'

Well, it did work a bit at first but one night I was sitting up watching the TV and it was getting brighter and brighter and brighter and all of a sudden there was a curl of smoke coming out of the back, so I turned it off straight away.

The next day I said, 'Your mate's done a fine thing. My television caught on fire!'

'Oh,' he said, 'I'll send him up to you again.'

The chap came up the next night.

'Oh,' he said, 'it's not too bad. It's a good job you didn't chuck the tea pot at it. That's what most people do. You just switched it off to let it settle down.'

So he put that right but I never got a good picture so I complained to the electric light company and they said,

'I'll tell you what, we'll put in a meter to read it,' and the meter showed that the power was going down which is why we had to have a booster at the bottom of the road, in about 1958.

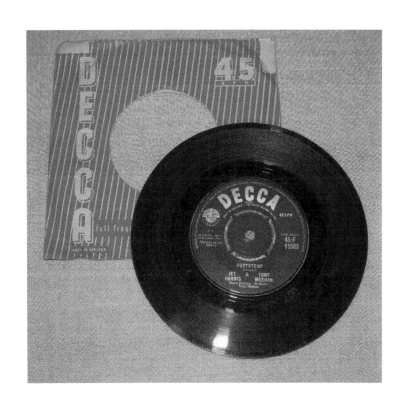

The Birth of the Single

1959

In '59 Decca wanted to give me a pension but I would lose money that way, because pensioned staff didn't do any overtime, so my twenty pounds a week was going to go down to about fifteen.

'I'll tell you what,' he said, 'You can have the time off in lieu. Instead of coming in at eight o'clock in the morning, come in at nine.'

I said, 'That's not much good to me.'

The others said, 'Come on, we've all got to lose,' so I agreed in the end. Then we kept pressing for midweek overtime and in the end we got it. I think the manager was only getting seven hundred a year and I was getting eight hundred because I put in a lot of hours and did weekend work too. We used to have to change over once a week. That meant you had to go in at 1 o'clock on Sunday afternoon right round to Monday morning. Going back the other way you went from seven o'clock on Saturday night and off at one o'clock Sunday.

In the meantime this seven inch record had come in called singles. We used to have a release every week but the timing was haphazard. Of course, all the kids wanted the record immediately they heard the song on the radio and they went to the shop but were disappointed 'cos it wasn't there. As you can imagine, if the kids couldn't get it at the time the song came out, then they'd forget about it because the next one'd be out. So in the end Decca gave them a release date.

'It will be in the shops on Monday morning,' they announced.

So that's how we came to have a weekly release. Everybody knew the new release would be there on that date which was a big boost for the industry.

That's when all the bands came in. HMV had the Beatles and we had The Rolling Stones. We had Freddy and the Dreamers too; I can't remember all the others but there were solo singers at that time too. Then of course these groups as good as did away with the solo singers like Val Doonican and Michael Holliday. Vera Lynn and Kathy Kirby both had their own shows on TV.

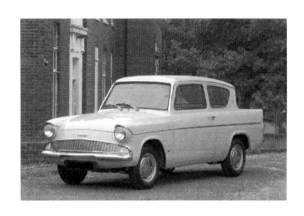

Ford Anglia 1960

1960

Mae's younger sister Gladys, who lived over the road from me, had married a fellow called Fred Wilby. His brother worked at Parnells before the war, where I worked making gun turrets for Wellington bombers back in 1938.

One day Fred said, 'My brother says he knows you.'
I said to Fred, 'How's Mae getting on.'
'Oh she's up in the Midlands. Yes she's doing all right.'
So I said, 'Good luck to her.'

So I thought she'd moved up there, so from then on I thought she was in the Midlands, but she was actually just visiting her daughter Jean.

1962

In 1962 I bought another new car, an Anglia. It was a new design where the window sloped at the back. I had that for two years and I got half the price for it when I traded it in for another Anglia. So after that I kept my car up to date by changing it every couple of years. Of course, as you went on you had to have two reflectors put on the back. Anglia's were dying out and so I went on to Escorts in 1965.

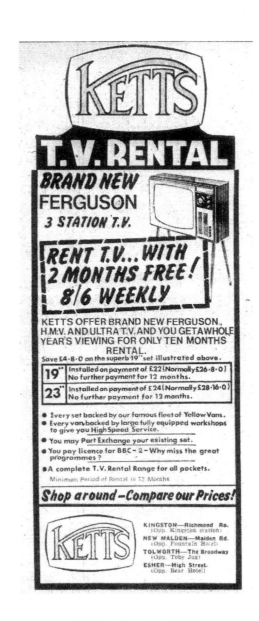

TV advert in 1969

Late 60's

Then colour TV came in. I bought a Decca set and it was so heavy. I thought, if I drop this there's all the money gone west. I got it home safely anyway, but I'd also sent away for an aerial. I had Pegg down here, and I was up in the loft twisting it about and she shouted, 'Yes, that's it!' So I fixed the aerial up there and we had a good picture for fourteen years.

I lost my picture at one time and I got a bloke round and he said,
    'You've got something in front of the aerial. You've got to go higher. You'll have to have it outside.'
    What had happened was these tall buildings had blocked the signal. The aerial had to go up once more but the next time he said that it was up as high as it could go. I had my snooker on one evening, that's my favourite sport, and there was a shadow; you had ten red balls and ten white balls so this bloke was up on the roof for about an hour and I remember it was a very cold day. I don't know how he stuck it up there.

    'I can't get a picture at all,' he said. 'You'll have to buy another aerial and I'll switch it to Guildford.' Then that was fine.

I got this new set and I said to the bloke,
    'What about the aerial?'
    'Don't worry about that. It's gone back the other way now.'
Of course I had to have a new aerial for this digital one last year too.
    I said, 'What about those tall buildings?'
    'That'll go through anything,' he said.

So that was my television history.

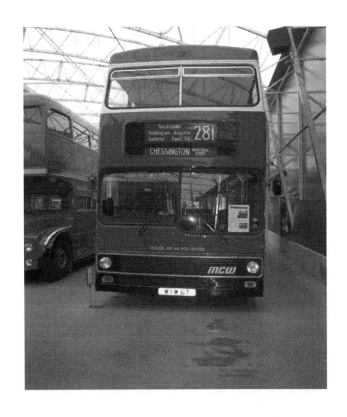

281
1970's bus to Surbiton

CHAPTER 25

Chance Encounters

1964

MY DAD LIVED for nine years after we moved in, 'til '64. Then I took over from him and I had a little bit more responsibility I suppose. I was doing it in those last years, collecting rent from next door. Rent was restricted for a while and things were going up and up, so they brought out a rule saying how much you could put the rent up. Up 'til then it had been £1 a week for donkeys' years.

Early 70's

Quite a while afterwards, I had another dog called Flash. Well, Mae always dressed smartly and do you know what, she always looked great in a hat. One day I was walking the dog and I remember thinking, that's quite a nice looking lady coming along here. She caught my eye as she passed and then I knew who it was. Oh, that's one of the Edwards, blimey that's Mae! Oh she must live around here now, I thought.

Years later I saw her again, walking across the road. I was taking some Christmas cards around locally and I bumped into her visiting her mother. It was dark and she was going home.

'Oh,' she said, 'I'm still up at The Ace.'

I said, 'I didn't know you were up The Ace.'

'Yes,' she said, 'Might see something of you.'

'Oh yes, Happy Christmas.' I said. I was so surprised because I thought she was still up in the Midlands.

The Ace of Spades was a night club, actually, and it's now a garage, but it's still called The Ace of Spades petrol station. She lived in the road opposite called Haycroft, so from then on I saw quite a bit of her because she was up and down there to her mother's. I saw quite a bit of her brother and sisters out of the window, too; and Gordon, I saw all of the family and that's how it went on.

She was always there, popping up.

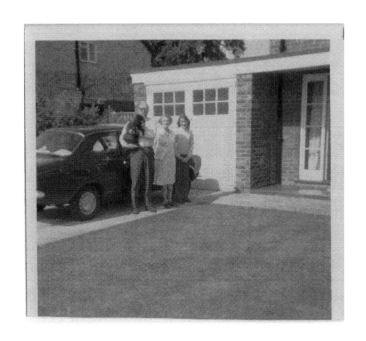

We had a poodle by then and we brought her when we came to see your family, Diana 11. Your Dad didn't like him so we tied him to the leg of a chair. Here is Peggy and I on one of our visits to St Albans with our poodle Susie.

11. Note that 'you' and 'your' is the compiler of this memois Diana Jackson

CHAPTER 26

The Final Decca Years

1972

AT DECCA THE brother of the man on nights was the foreman and when he died I got made up to foreman but I said I don't want any nights. I think I had the flu at that time and the other chap who was a foreman came over and said,

'They've made us an offer. We can change month about but we'll be paid overtime rates day and night.'

So I thought that'd only be forty four hours and there'd be no need to do any overtime.

'Think about it,' he said.

So I thought, I've only got eighteen months to go and so I agreed.

1974

We were just experimenting with the CD at Decca just before I left in '74. I was there for thirty seven years and left earning £168 a month net, with all the tax and everything taken off; a lousy sum really.

When I retired I used to busy myself doing things like building the cupboard upstairs and doing things in the shed and I took over the decorating too. We went away to hotels in the end and we went to Bournemouth a few times.

In '74 your family were at St Albans Diana, and I bought an orange Escort and I thought, that's my last car. We used to break 'em in in those days, so I said,

'Right, we'll go to St Albans.'

So week after week we came to St Albans to see you all.

1975/76

Penny our poodle died and one Sunday morning Pegg went down the road for a paper. She got chatting to a bloke and he had this white poodle and wondered if we could find a home for it. Pegg brought it home.

I said, 'No more dogs!'

Pegg said, 'Go on, it's a nice one.'

I didn't often win an argument with Pegg! I put my foot down sometimes but usually I went along with it. We didn't have the poodle for long because it died and it's buried at the top of the garden. No more dogs after that.

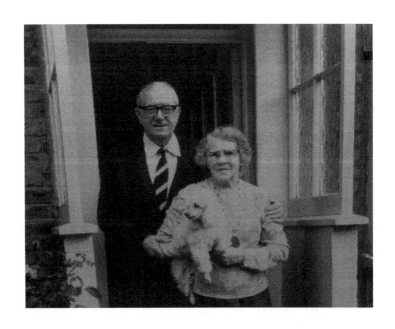

Norman and Peggy at home

1978

Peggy must have been 80 when she passed away. She was ten years older than me of course, but she never had a birth certificate. We tried to get her one for her pension but she hadn't been registered. Apparently in those days you didn't have to, I don't know, but anyway they couldn't find her birth certificate so we couldn't get a pension. In the end, during the war we were issued with an Identity Card and they said,

'If you've got an Identity Card, we'll issue it from there.'

I lost Pegg in 1978. She had a brain haemorrhage. I made her a cup of tea and took it upstairs; I always made her a cup in the mornings. She was putting her stockings on and then she fell back and she went all shaky.

'Oh God,' I said. 'What's up with you?'

She'd gone. That was a bit of a shock that was.

I shouted, 'Don't go Pegg, don't leave me, don't leave me!'

We had forty one years together. That's not bad is it?

You used to call us Mr and Mrs Campbell, right up to when Peggy died. After Pegg died your mother said,

'We can't go on like this anymore, we must call you Norman.'

I get the same with Jock's family in Scotland. He was one of our lodgers too, like your father. Now Myra, she's 68, and she's a grandma but she still calls me Uncle Norman, because her mother had instilled it in her. One of her children is a doctor now and she still calls me Uncle Norman and so do their children.

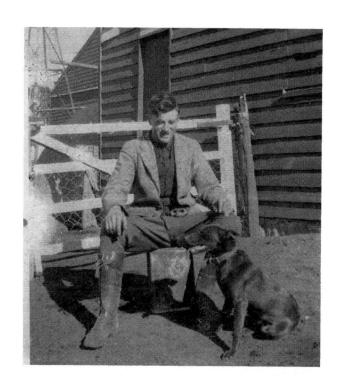

Mae had this photo of Norman in her handbag for fifty years!

CHAPTER 27

Childhood Sweethearts Unite!

1979

IN 1976 MAE had lost her husband but I didn't know about that until I met up with another old pal, Bill, who I sometimes visited at his place up in Chessington. Pegg and I went up there quite a bit and then I went on my own because Pegg had just died in 1979.

One day he said, 'Did you know that Mae's lost her husband and is on her own now and she still lives at Haycroft?'

'Well, no I didn't,' I replied, 'I'll have to take a look down there one day,' and I laughed, because I was on my own now too.

Before I could do that Mae had heard that I'd lost Pegg but Gladys her sister had said, 'You're not to go down there.'

Anyway, every Friday or Saturday she used to come up to see Gladys, who lived over the road. One day she came but Gladys wasn't in and so she had an idea. I'll go over and ask Norman if I can borrow a wheelbarrow.

'Come on in,' I said. 'I knew you were there before you even knocked.' Strange wasn't it. The wheelbarrow was just an excuse. (Norman laughed)

From then on that was it. It was just like we'd been together all our lives. (Norman got a little emotional at this point) It gelled right from the beginning and it felt just like family.

Before that another woman down the road rang me up and asked me out to dinner, but I thought, I'm not having any of that. So I said, 'No sorry,' and so she got talking to Mae and so Mae said that her first thoughts were, I'll make sure I'm up there first!

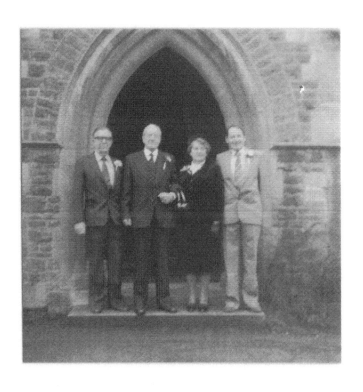

Mae and I waited 60 years for this moment!

After all those years!

When Mae and I got together again, we were seventy years old and she surprised me when she said,

'I've still got that snapshot of you. I've carried it in my handbag since you went to Australia.'.... Unbelievable.

She said, 'That's the only safe place, because my husband, he might have got jealous, so I hid it deep down and I've carried it all these years.'

That's a place no one is ever going to look, in her handbag so there you are. (Norman chuckled)

Mae and Norman

Christmas Eve 1979

'It's a bit sudden,' they said, 'With Pegg just gone.'

I said, 'Well, she's gone and there's nothing I can do to bring her back.'

I thought, well, I'm seventy years of age. I may only have five years. Why wait?

We had seventeen years actually. I married Mae on Christmas Eve 1979 about eighteen months after Pegg died. I met lots of Mae's family that day. There was Mae's eldest daughter Jean and her husband David and they brought their two sons over from America, Nigel and Guy, but their daughter didn't come because she was married.

Then there was Trevor and his wife Margaret and their daughter Dena from Jersey, and Michael and his two children Debbie and Paul. Then there was Graham and Janet and their four children. Micheal was local from Raynes Park and Janet and Graham were from Chessington. You see, I met most of Mae's family at our wedding. Then there was Roger and his wife Marian from Jersey and Sandra from Australia but they couldn't come.

It was a very special day. It felt just right somehow but It's hard to describe how I felt.

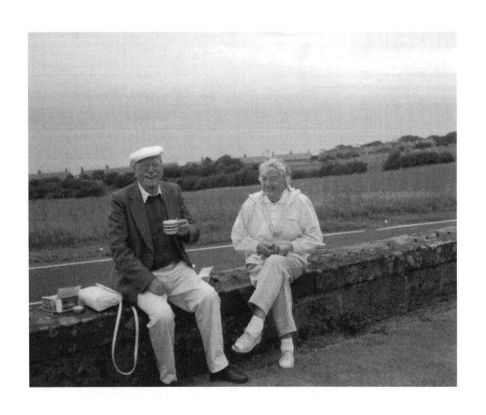

Enjoying a picnic in harmony.

The 1980's

The rest of the family raised the money for Sandra and her husband to come over from Australia in the October of 1980. Then I'd met all the family except Roger and Marian, which must have been in 1981 when they came from Jersey with their two children a year later. So that's how I met all the family and I got on alright with them all. They were all pleased for us and we've had good relations ever since.

We lived life to the full, Mae and I. She had a big family and so we'd have days out visiting them. Gwen, Mae's sister had a little place down in Shoreham in Kent; a lovely little village and we went down there quite a bit. Then we used to go to Wynn's down at Seven Oaks. All of the sisters were alive so they used to go out with us. There was also Mae's brother Gordon and his wife. We were doing fine for company.

'I'm glad you've come into the family,' Gordon's wife said. 'You're the only brother in law we've got now.' Because you see they'd all lost their husbands, the four sisters, but Gordon was still married to his wife. There was Gwyn, Olive, Mae, Gordon and Gladys, five of them.

We went over to Jersey several times but I never stayed with any of them. They've been here but we always stayed in a hotel or Bed and Breakfast. There was a good one just at the bottom of the next street from Trevor's house in St Helier. Roger lives the other end of the island in St Mary's so they came down to see us at Trevor's place. Marian worked in a shoe shop in St Helier.

Then Jean, she came over every year from America but at first David didn't come because he was working, but when they retired they said they'd come every three months if we'd have them.

'Of course we'll have you,' we said. Then it got down to more or less once a year.

When David and Jean came over we used to hire a car because I wouldn't let anyone else drive my car. We used to go all over the country and Bed and Breakfast. We went to Scotland, North Wales, South Wales, in fact all over Wales. We stayed in York and Chester and radiated out from there.

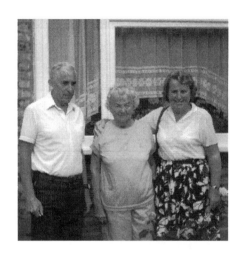

Mae with Pat and Arthur 12

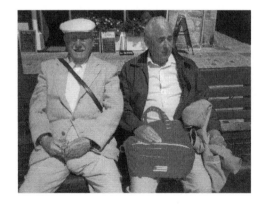

Norman and Arthur

12 Pat and Arthur Jackson. Diana Jackson's parents

We also went to the West Country of course, right down to Penzance, Lands End and all around Cornwall, along the South Coast to Christchurch and Bournemouth and down to Weymouth and Oakhampton. That was in the first ten years with Mae. Unfortunately in the last seven years she wasn't well.

Mae and Janet were always very close even before I came into the family and she was always popping in and of course Mae used to go baby-sitting. They were pretty thick because they were the only ones really close in Haycroft. I was up in Haycroft one day and Mae said, 'You answer it.' So that was the first time I spoke to Janet over the phone.

When we were married we saw a lot of Michael from Raynes Park near Wimbledon. Of course when Trevor and Margaret came over or Marian we'd have them all over here on a Sunday afternoon and Michael used to come over to do odd jobs for us. A handyman he is.

It was funny because there was always washing out on the line.
    I said, 'How do we always get pictures of us when all the washing's on the line!'
We used to have quite a few get togethers at one time or another.

We saw lots of friends too. We even went on holiday with Pat and Arthur, your Mum and Dad.

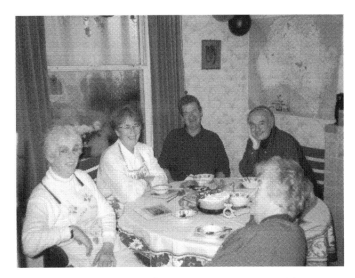

Jean, Sandra, Richard, David and Mae

Mae's family

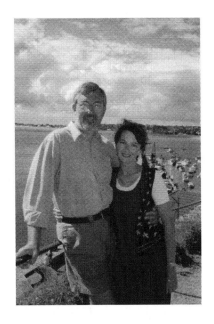

Philip and Dena

Family in Jersey

Jersey

1996 to 1998

Then of course we had these trips over to Jersey on a Friday night for ten pounds. We'd get over there on Saturday morning and go up to Trevor's for a while and have our breakfast and have a look round the town. Then Roger would come down and we'd have a chat with them. Then they'd all come down and see us off on the boat at midnight, or just before, and we'd sail back to Weymouth, getting in at about eleven o'clock Sunday morning.

We'd get two bottles of wine and a bottle of whiskey all in the ten pounds. That wasn't bad was it? So we went about four times.

Australia again

1988

Mae's daughter Sandra went to Australia years ago with her family and then they went to New Zealand. She met Richard in the Union Office and they got married. He came over here and he was a nice fellow and went to the college up the top of the road. Then they came over here together at Christmas and Jean and David were here too. We did have a good time that Christmas and New Year in about 1988.

They were surprised to hear that I'd been to Australia too and so when they went back home they went exploring where I was in the 1920's. They met the Brown family where I stayed in Cope Cope and they also went to the museum in Donald.

I gave Richard a few things to take with them including my passport and my steamer ticket. I never gave it up at the end of my trip you see, I don't know why, but he took them to the museum and they appreciated it. They gave him some copies of articles which they brought back to me.

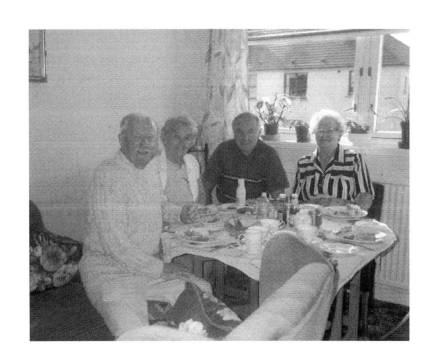

Norman and Mae visiting Agnes and Jock in Scotland.
Jock was one of Norman and Peggy's first lodgers who
stayed with them in Kingston during WW2

1989

It was my 80th birthday and we went to Scotland in one of my Escorts. On the way back we always used to do one hundred miles and have a break, then do another one hundred miles and have another break and so on, but on the third break we broke down, so I thought I'd go over to the garage I could see.

'What do you want to do that for? You're in the AA,' Mae said.

So I called the AA up and we had to wait for them to come out for a couple of hours but when the man arrived he said,

'What's happened sir is that your alternator cable has been cut. In the alternator cable there are seven cables and you've cut through two of them. I can bind it up together to get you home.'

So I said, 'OK.'

By this time it was dark and I didn't like driving at night. It must have been midnight or one o'clock in the morning so I thought, oh well, we'd better start off, so I went down the motorway, but no sooner had we got started that we came to road works. Then I looked at the sign and we were on the M5 and not the M6. I was on the wrong road. You know you can't turn round so we had to keep on going.

Then there were signs up about the Severn Bridge and so I thought, how far off am I? Then I saw a sign for Oxford but I didn't know my way so I thought, keep going, keep going. Finally I'd had enough! So I turned into a service station and we waited until it got light but we couldn't sleep. You saw all the cars coming and going; vehicles broken down and being towed away. A lot went on while we were sitting there. At seven o'clock in the morning we set off again. Of course I could see where we were then, so we got on to the M4 and we were home in no time. We went into Sainsbury's, did a bit of shopping and we were home at nine o'clock. That was a terrible night.

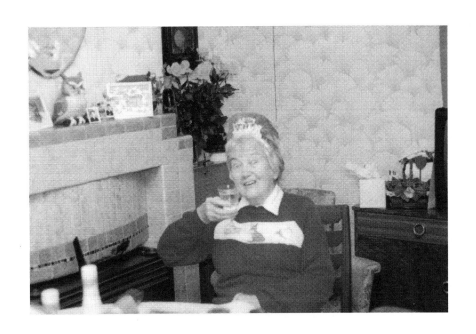

Happy Christmas at home

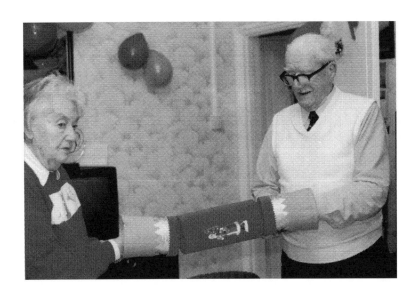

1990's

For the first ten years we got on like a house on fire, Mae and I, but in the last seven years Mae had this disease called Shingles. The old wives tale is that if it goes all round you, you're supposed to die. It was very painful and she had it up on her shoulders and it blistered so that you couldn't touch her.

In the car she'd exclaim, 'Can't you go any slower,' because she could feel any little bump.

'I can't go any slower darling,' I used to say.

They gave her pain killers but she wouldn't take them because they'd make her dizzy. It frightened her that it might turn her brain, because her father, he had Alzheimer's, so understandably she wasn't very happy in the last seven years.

I was seventeen years with Mae; not bad was it. I was forty one years with Peggy then I've had twelve to thirteen on my own. It's been the loneliness I've found hard to cope with. Having somebody all those years and now nobody. That's what gets me and I wonder what it's all about.

Mae was taken bad on Boxing Day 1996 and David and Jean were over. She was taken to hospital and we waited all day for news, pacing the corridors until at about 10 o'clock the doctor said,

'You can take your wife home now.'

I said, 'She's only in her nightdress. She's not in a fit state to go home, so she stayed in overnight.

The next day we went to see her and she had a black eye. She'd fallen out of bed because they hadn't put up the guard. She wasn't very well at all.

'Get me out of here' she said.

'I can't do that darling,' I said.

Some days she was a bit better but one afternoon I sat with her and suddenly she sat bolt upright in bed with her hands stretched out in front of her. Then she settled back down to sleep. Later that evening David came to stay with her but he was usually home by 8 o'clock. He arrived home at 10 o'clock and she'd gone.

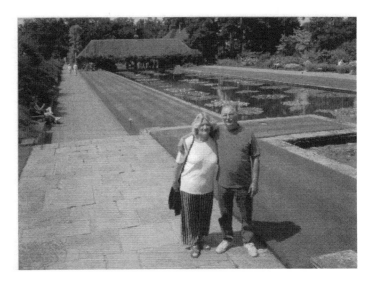

Janet and Graham at RHS Wisley Gardens
I don't know what I would have done without Mae's family

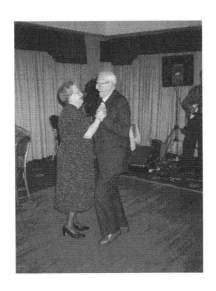

I also went up to Scotland for Agnes's birthday in 1998

CHAPTER 28

Without Mae

1996 to 2000

MAE AND I had always been together. You get accustomed to having someone around all the time but then you get left hours and hours on your own.

When Mae died there was no one to take out and I didn't want to go out on my own. This is no good, going down to Brighton and sitting on my own, I thought. It was useless. I'd sooner walk into Surbiton. My car was standing there doing nothing costing me thirty quid a week so I got rid of it. So I sold it to Bill Underhill in Scotland for his son. He was working down here at that time so he drove it back up. I had that car for ten years.

All the big families in the area had gone now too. I knew everybody and now I know nobody. What happened?

Since Mae died I've been so many hours on my own. You get a bit down in the dumps sometimes and wonder. What's it all about, because it was just a blank really. What's tomorrow for? Just to eat and drink. What's tomorrow, to eat and drink the same.

It was really hard but I was lucky though. When I got Mae everybody else came with her! I had no family of my own before Mae and all her family have kept in touch since she died. Michael still rings a lot and I talk to Jean in America. They all correspond even now. I went over to Jersey for Wayne, Roger's son's wedding in 2000. Jean, David Janet, and Graham came over too.

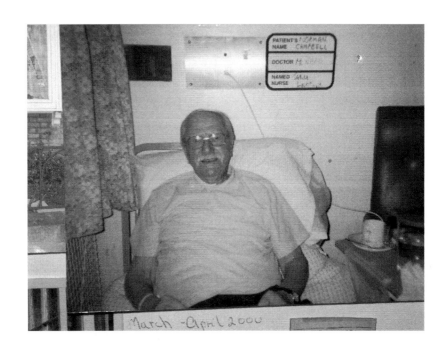

Recovering from Heart Surgery
Aged 91 years

CHAPTER 29

Back from the Brink

2000

I don't know what I would have done without Graham and Janet when I was ill in 2000 and in hospital. They were my lifeline and I don't know what would have happened otherwise.

It all started with a terrible back ache and eventually I thought I'd better call the doctor. She came and Janet and Graham came too.

'But I came to see you about a back ache some months ago,' the doctor said.

'But this is a different kind of back ache,' I said.

She got me to stretch up and she ran her fingers down my back and she said, 'I think I'd better send you for a scan.'

'What, go to hospital tonight?' I asked.

'Yes,' she said.

Suddenly all the blood seemed to run down from my head and I was gone. They had to get an ambulance and away we went. We got to Kingston but they had no one who could treat me and so I got transferred to Hammersmith.

'We've got a team all waiting,' they said.

'But he's 91,' Graham said.

'That's all right. We do them all ages. Wheel him in,' he said.

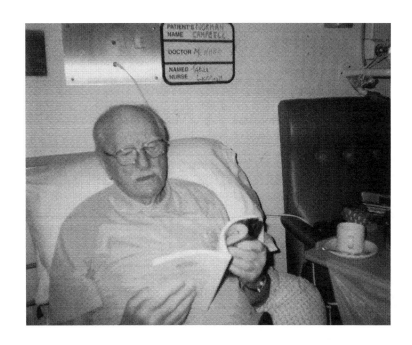

Getting Better!

I was in surgery for I don't know how many hours but it was 2 o'clock in the morning and Janet was still at the hospital.

'Can we see him,' she asked.

Graham went in and he said there were wires and blood all over the place.

'You looked terrible,' he told me, so he asked the doctor,

'What are his chances?'

'Well,' the doctor replied. 'We've done all we can. It's up to him now. If he's here in the morning he is, and if he's not, he's not. That's his chances!'

Then at Hammersmith Hospital they said,

'We've got no intensive care.'

So I was wheeled off to St Thomas's where I was watched every day and night for a fortnight. They pumped so many drugs in me that I when I came too I was hallucinating. I thought I'd been in a car accident.

Then they sent me back to Hammersmith for a fortnight but while I was in the ambulance I asked the nurse about the accident.

'You weren't in a car accident,' she said. 'You had an aorta embolism.'

'What's that?' I said.

'Your main artery burst,' she explained.

I'm not sure but I think they had my heart all out on the side while they tried to mend the artery!

Once at Hammersmith they decided to arrange rehabilitation and they sent me to Tolworth. I ended up there for another six weeks. I made quite a few friends in there and they say I'm a bit of a miracle.

Surrey Comet

SC   OCTOBER 2, 2009

OCT **2009**

the register

If you have an item for the editorial section of the Register – births, weddings, ot
contact David Rankin on 020 8330 9546 or drankin@london.newsquest.co.uk

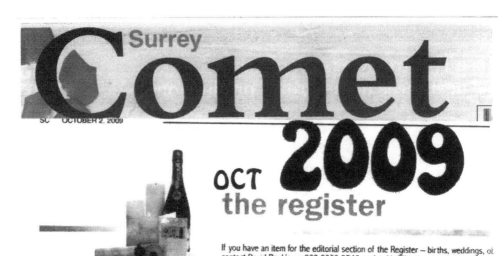

100th birthday: Norman Campbell

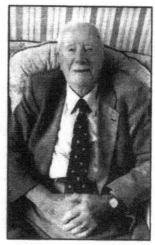

Family party: Norman Campbell

With the impressive sound system sitting in Norman Campbell's front room, it is fair to say he is not your typical 99-year-old.

But Norman, who turns 100 on Sunday, loves his music and does not need any help from youngsters to put on his favourite CDs.

His taste in music has not changed, with him still insisting the 20s and 30s were the best, but his house has changed beyond recognition from when he first moved in at the age of two.

Back then, there was only one tap in the house, no bathroom and not a thing was wasted.

He can still recall the Depression, when things got so bad that his family were all out of work and living off just 13 shillings.

He said: "You'd buy a newspaper for a penny and you'd use it for everything – toilet paper, wrapping paper, to cover the table, the lot.

"There's no recession now – the road is full of cars and the shops are filled with people. You can't make people understand that, they have no idea."

Although Mr Campbell never had any children with his first wife Peggy, to whom he was married for 41 years, he now counts six children, 15 grandchildren, 15 great-grandchildren and one great-great-grandchild as his own.

In a love story to warm the heart, he recalled how he came to have such a large brood thanks to a woman he refers to as "my May".

He said: "May was six and I was five and we went to school together. We ended up pairing off together, we just sort of gelled."

It ended when he went to Australia, where he spent some time sheep farming from the age of 18.

He spent four years there and, when he came back, May had married. When he spotted her in the street she said: "You better not be seen talking to me, I'm a mother with a husband."

Years later, after both of their partners had died, there was a knock at Norman's door – it was May.

Norman married her within a year, on Christmas Eve, at the age of 70, and inherited her extensive family.

May died in 1997 but all of her children will be there for Norman for a big party in Chessington on Saturday.

Norman hopes to enjoy many more as well.

He said: "I might live to 120. Well, you never know, do you?"

❏ **Turning 100? Tell us at surreycomet.co.uk/news**

CHAPTER 28

100 yr Celebration

4th October 2009

I HAVE FAMILY all over the world now and they were at my 100th birthday. All were family except Myra and Bill from Scotland and the lady next door.

My 100th birthday took a lot of organising which was all down to Janet. It all started with somebody I've never had anything to do with before called Nigel, Jean's eldest son, who said one day,

'We want to go over for Norman's 100th birthday.'

He started it and that was that. He also says that he'll come over for my 105th so we've got to get ready for that now.

So in January of the year 2009 Janet said,

'Shall we see who's coming?'

You see they had to take time off from work and Jean and David said they'd bring all their family from America.

Trevor and his wife, daughter and her two boys, they came from Jersey. Michael and Val came, but not their children. There was Graham and his four children, three of whom are married so they all came with their children. Graham, Roger and Marian, they came. Then there was Sandra and Chris and her daughter and children, they came too and also my Great Grandchildren from Australia.

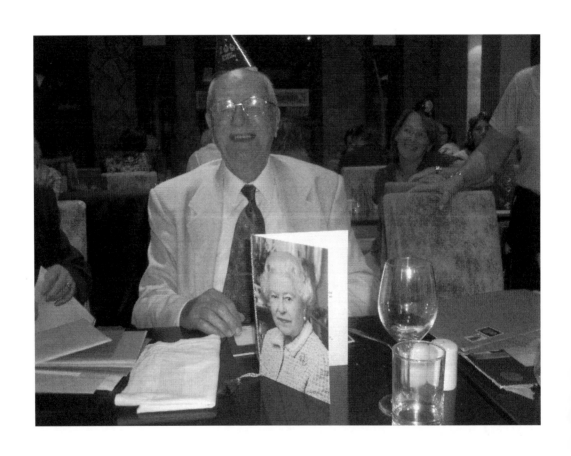

Greetings from the Queen

We said we'd have to book up a hotel and the best one round our way is the Holiday Inn, next door to Chessington. It would be a good place to hold it because they could get busses and trains from there. We arranged it in July and I got the rooms all booked up when I went up there and sorted it all out with the reception. Janet had all these people from all over the world meeting at this hotel. That was absolutely remarkable. It was a grand night. I got them all together like that. I mean they'd never all got together before. Unbelievable!

We had two other couples, Barbara and Sid and Myra and Bill who were two outsiders. Myra is the daughter of Jock, one of my first lodgers, just like your father was an early lodger. We had a party on the Saturday evening, which was the third actually. I was all against that because it was not my birthday which was on the 4th, but Janet said,

'I can't get all my lot there on the Sunday because they've got to go to work on the Monday,' so it had to be on the Saturday.

'I know,' I said. 'I'm going to see if I can get a bus and get them all up to the Claygate Centre for Sunday lunch too,' so I enquired of the manageress.

'Yes,' she said, 'but you have to get the cake in and see that all the catering's done.'

I didn't want to worry about all that so I asked Janet what she thought and she said, 'Well, they do hold a carvery at the hotel on a Sunday and they'd give you half of the place to yourself.'

So I agreed, but we also asked all those who didn't come on the Saturday night to join us on the Sunday too. Of course your father, he said,

'I'll just pop over to say Happy Birthday to you on the Sunday.' I had a job to get him to come to lunch so I said,

'Bring Diana [13] and Roger,' and so he did. The next door neighbours have been good to me so I asked them too.

13. That's me, the compiler!

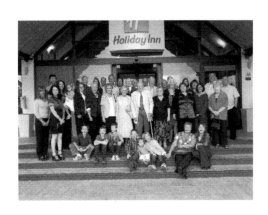

Celebrating with all my
Family

We had a buffet on the Saturday evening. They stayed up until about two to three o'clock in the morning. Of course we moved out of the room into a bar and they all had a good time. I had hired the room for £400 and we had a buffet. Quite nice though.

Guy's wife, who I'd never met before, had an idea. The last time I'd met Guy was for the wedding when he was only fourteen. He hadn't been over since and of course he's married now and he must be forty odd, I don't know. Anyway, she was keen on getting all that rhyming slang. Everyone was trying to remember them all and she was writing them down.

'Oh yes,' shouted someone, 'Up the Frog and Toad!'
'Apples and Pears.'
'Yes we've got that.'
'Mince pies.'
'Oh yes.'
So there was quite a bit of fun going on. I bought them a round of drinks to start with and a round of drinks at midnight to wish me a Happy Birthday and I bought a round of drinks on the Sunday before we had dinner. Me, Jean and David came back here just after midnight.

'I'd better make a move,' I said. 'Otherwise I'll be here all night.' I had thought I'd come back here about 9 o'clock you know, but I stayed there until after twelve!

It was a great success.

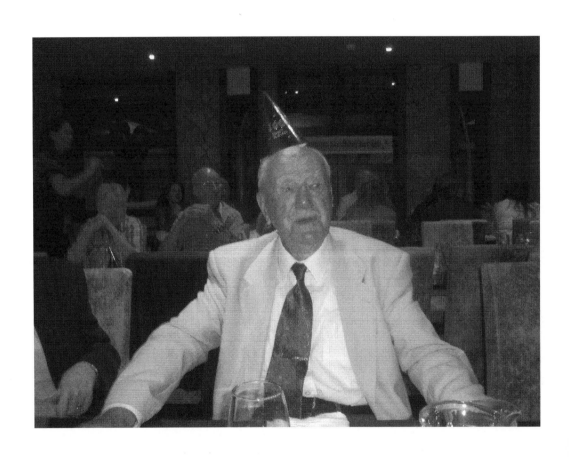

Never too old to Celebrate!

100 YEARS Old Today!

4th October 1909 to 4th October 2009

On the Sunday we had the carvery and there were speeches and all these photos were taken. Philip turned up with his camera and he took lots. Dina from Jersey had put together a sheet all about my life to give out and we had party hats with 100 on them.

It was great wasn't it?

I had no family before Mae and now I've got all this lot. There were over 40 people there. Unbelievable!

2009 - 2011
Strange thing about it was, do you know how many I had for my 101st? One!
Then for my 102nd? Two!'

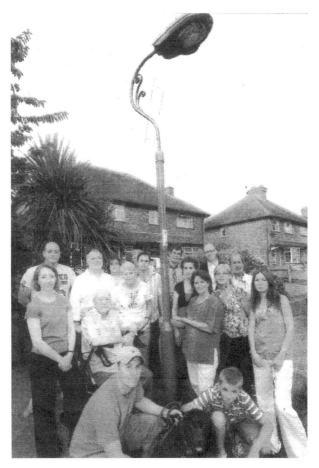

Getting Involved with the Community

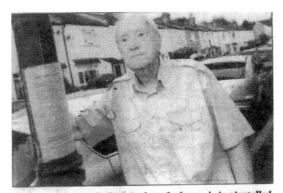

Norman Campbell remembers the lamps being installed.

CHAPTER 29

Life Goes On

The Victorian Street Lamps and the Local Paper

2010

Since then my neighbours said we're going to hold a meeting down at the pub about the street lamps. Surrey County Council had said that they had to replace the old lighting. They put a sample down the bottom of the road which started it all off.

Everyone said they wanted to keep their old Victorian street lamp, because it gave character to the street. There was a petition and a council representative came who explained,

'It would cost £4,000 for each lamp if they took them down, cleaned them up and restored them or £2,000 for replacement imitation lamps with swan necks, much like the old ones, which were Edwardian incidentally and not Victorian. I know because I was here when they put them up. They were gas lamps in those days of course. The road was built in 1904, the gas lamps put in in 1914 and electricity lamps didn't come in until 1932.

Well, after the meeting everyone agreed to raise the £2,000. A photo was taken of me next to one of the old lamps and it was put in the paper. I had to look cross. I didn't really mind what they did but it was a nice chance to get to know some of the neighbours. They didn't come back to ask me to contribute for the new lamps though.

Since my birthday people have taken more notice of me, I think, and now I've got this woman coming in here, a companion, and I think it'll make a difference. Thinking about you writing about my life; that's good too. It gives me something to look forward to. When you start asking me questions it starts to bring it all out.

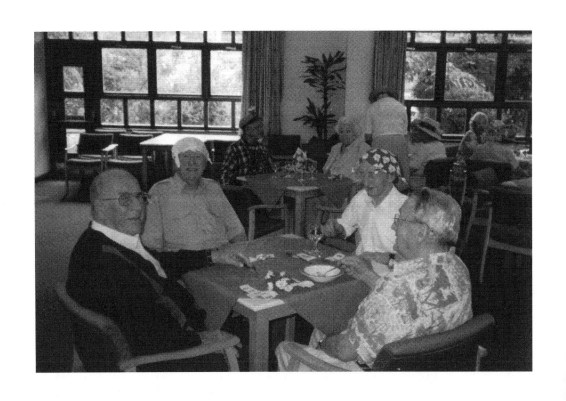

Having Fun at the Mayfield Avenue Centre

Old Friends and New!

2011

Just last week I met a lady from Mayfield Avenue who likes to have a jaw. I went down to the club one Thursday and as I went in to pay for my dinner she came up and said, 'hello.'

'You don't generally come on a Thursday,' I said.

'No I'm up here to meet a friend, a new member. I'm just showing her the ropes,' she said.

So that was that. I went away and when I came back all the people were sitting around waiting to go into the dining room, so of course I passed them both.

'Oh,' she said. 'This is my friend I told you about. She comes from Rectory Lane.'

'Oh, Rectory Lane, that sounds interesting.' I said this because there might be somebody down the line. Not in my age limit, but someone down the line. I always think I'm going to meet somebody like that; the next generation. My generation's gone of course.

'I said, 'How long have you been living in Rectory Lane?'

'Nineteen years,' she said.

'That's only yesterday,' I said. 'I shan't know anybody you know.'

So I sat down in the dining room waiting for all the people filling up and these two made a bee line and sat with me. We still talked of Rectory Lane.

'In the Elms we had a swimming bath,' she said.

'Oh, you know about the swimming baths.'

'Yes, they had a swimming bath in the Elms,' she said.

'I know that,' I said. 'It was started off as a pond with two Elm trees and we asked the man in charge, Mr Clayton, if we could have a swimming bath. We were always asking for something or other and he said yes. If you start digging it up I'll finish it off. So that's how the swimming bath started.'

She knows about the swimming bath I thought.

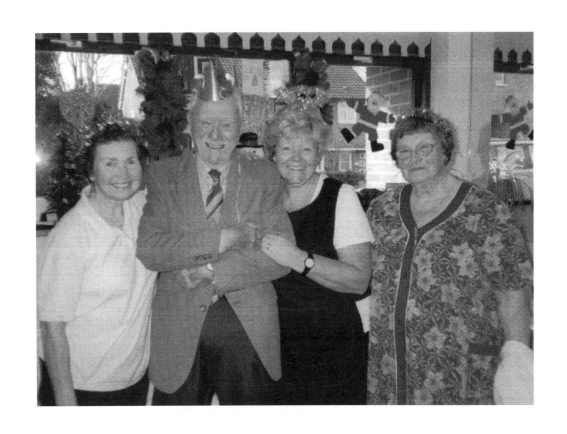

Christmas Celebrations!

Then we talked about Aunt Sally, which was a cut through from Rectory Lane to Ditton Hill Road.

I said, 'Harts lived in there and Skiptons on the other side.'

'No, the Chataulphs lived there. They rented it off of Harts,' she said.

'That's later,' I said, 'but what I know is that Harts lived in that house and the Gibsons in the next one.'

'Well, my father in law was a police constable.'

'What was his name?'

'Berry.'

'Berry!' I said. 'I know you husband. Stan. We used to go to school together.'

So now I've now met somebody I can talk to about my days.

She started off in Tolworth and then she lived in Ditton Hill Road. When they built houses at the other end of Rectory Lane they lived in one of those and I was the same age as her husband.

'When did Stan die?' I asked.

'Thirty seven years ago,' she said.

'You didn't get any pension then.' She was a bit grieved about that.

'Never mind,' I said. 'I've been drawing some of his for the last thirty seven years!'

Stan's father was a policeman. At that time they had police constables all over the place. There were thirteen just up this road. Of course the Police Stations were in the little villages; one in Tolworth, one in Claygate and one in Kingston. They were scattered all over the place. I knew Berry and I knew Amos, another policeman who lived lower down.

Well Stan, her husband, we went to school together and we were in the boys brigade at the same time too.

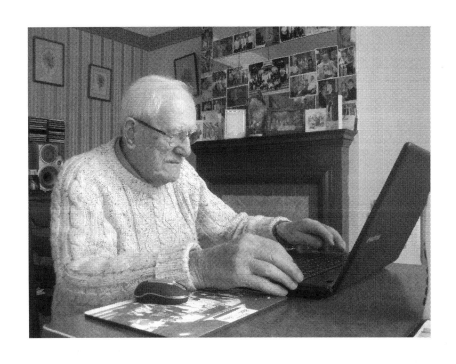

New Challenges @ 102 years

CHAPTER 30

A Very Silver Surfer at 102!

2012

Now Michael rings up every other day and his daughter Helen lives next door. Jean and David come over from America each year but I'm not sure about this year. Jean's now eighty so I'm not so sure if she's allowed to travel. She still works hard though, stacking wood for the winter. I speak to Jean every Sunday evening and I also speak to your Mum every Sunday morning too, at 10.30 on the dot.

I never went out there to America. They were always asking me to go. Jean tells everybody about me. The other day she said,

'I'm seeing a professor and I'm going to tell him that you've got a computer.'

I told Roger this week.

'Cor,' he said. 'You haven't! I'm amazed.' He said. 'I never thought he'd go up the pole over it. 'That's marvellous,' he said.

This is how it happened. One day, I had gone to the front door and there was this chap doing the glazing next door. We had quite a chat for a while. I told him I was 102 and of course he said,

'You can't be.'

I was telling him that I was stuck indoors all day long with only the walls to talk to. I get so lonely you see. I've got carers popping in but once they are gone I'm on my own again. I want somebody I can talk to, to stop the monotony.

He said, 'I know a carer; a friend of mine. I'll get her to get in touch with you.'

That's how it happened. I told her to come up and have an interview. She used to be in PR, going up to London everyday by train, but then she lost her mother and father in a car accident and it turned her whole life around and so she studied to be a carer. Now she comes in as a companion for me twice a week because when she came I moaned, 'I'm just lonely!'

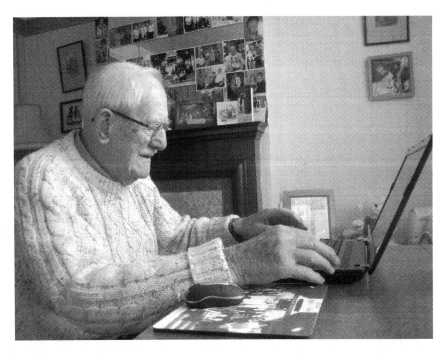

I Now Chat to Family and Friends on Skype

We had a chat and then she said,

'You're bright. You should get yourself a computer.'

'A computer!' I said. 'What would I want a computer for? I can't be bothered with that. They keep bombarding me with, 'Get on line, visit our website,' and all this on the television.

Susi said, 'I bought one from Sainsbury's for £279. Would you like me to get you one?'

I thought about it. Susi's here and I'm going to get a tutor for nothing; that's quick thinking. So I said, 'Yes, you do that.'

'Ok then. I'll go to Sainsbury's and get you one.'

She came back and said,

'This was only £239, £50 cheaper than mine!'

That's how it started. Of course I'm all right when she's here, but when I lose something she gets me out of it, but I'm getting better as it goes along. I go along with me typing and it should go back automatically but sometimes it doesn't, it stops, so I put it away and wait 'til Susi comes back. She says that it goes back automatically and so does Janet but sometimes it doesn't for me, so she said, 'Type it so far and then go back..'

'Wait a minute,' I said. 'Let's take a step at a time. I've got enough to get on with.'

Susi's ever such a nice person and there's a whole new world out there for me on my computer. She would do anything I ask her to but I make her laugh so that's good.

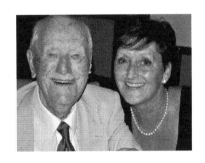

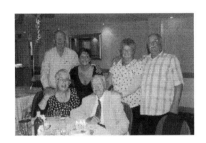

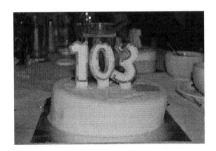

Snapshots of Norman's 103rd birthday

So that's what I do now when I'm on my own.

My computer has opened up a new world but it takes up all my time. I've got sixteen addresses now. I sent an email to Sandra in New Zealand and no sooner had I sent it but she sent one back. I'm on Skype too, where you can talk and see at the same time and I'm set up on Sainsbury's for shopping. All I have to do is press the button and I can shop. All these things you can do. Unbelievable! All the games you can play, too. If there's nothing on television I watch all my favourite big band tunes on YouTube and old comics too. There's so much.

There were six of us at my 103rd. Janet and Graham, Sandra and Chris and Susi, my carer. It was quite a day.

But sometimes I just want to be looked after though., all the time. Getting dressed takes me over an hour and making a cup of tea is sometimes just too much effort . Yes, I just want to be looked after now, so I've sorted it. Someone comes in every morning and every night I sit down exhausted because I just haven't got the strength anymore. I climb upstairs to the bathroom just to have some exercise. You want to do things in your head but you just can't, but I know that it's doing things for myself and keeping active that keeps me alive.

It's as simple as that!

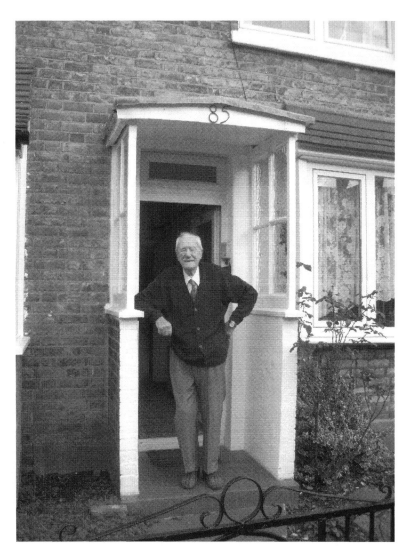

I moved here in 1911 and
I'm still here in 2012!

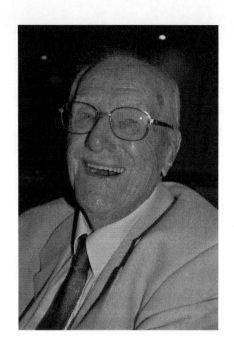

Norman @ 103 years

He passed away
only two months later on
9th December 2012

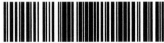

Made in the USA
Charleston, SC
13 May 2013